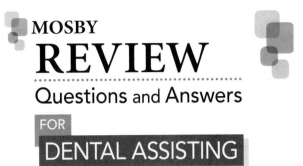

MOSBY
REVIEW
Questions and Answers

FOR
DENTAL ASSISTING

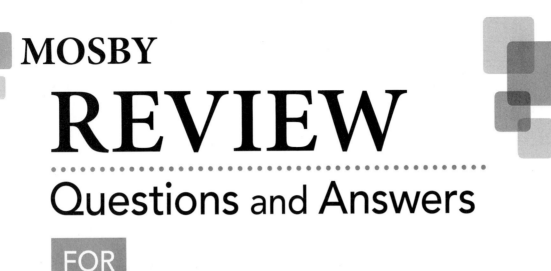

MOSBY
REVIEW
Questions and Answers
FOR
DENTAL ASSISTING

EDITED AND CONTRIBUTED BY

Betty Ladley Finkbeiner, RDA, MS

Faculty Emeritus
Washtenaw Community College
Ann Arbor, Michigan
Dental Assisting/Educational Consultant
Fort Myers, Florida

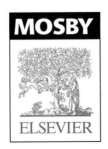

MOSBY

ELSEVIER

11830 Westline Industrial Drive
St. Louis, Missouri 63146

MOSBY REVIEW QUESTIONS AND ANSWERS FOR DENTAL ASSISTING   ISBN: 978-0-323-05284-9
Copyright © 2009 by Mosby, Inc., an affiliate of Elsevier Inc.

Notice

Neither the Publisher nor the Editors assume any responsibility for any loss or injury and/or damage to persons or property arising out of or related to any use of the material contained in this book. It is the responsibility of the treating practitioner, relying on independent expertise and knowledge of the patient, to determine the best treatment and method of application for the patient.

The Publisher

Library of Congress Control Number 2007941950

Senior Editor: John Dolan
Managing Editor: Jaime Pendill
Editorial Assistant: Joslyn Dumas
Publishing Services Manager: Melissa Lastarria
Project Manager: Mary Pohlman
Design Manager: Amy Buxton

Printed in United States of America

Last digit is the print number: 9 8 7 6 5 4 3 2 1

Contributors

Sharron J. Cook, CDA
Instructor, Dental Assisting
School of Health Sciences
Columbus Technical College
Columbus, Georgia

W. Stephen Eakle, DDS
Professor, Clinical Dentistry
Chief, Section of Patient Care
Division of General Dentistry
Department of Preventive and Restorative Dental
   Sciences
School of Dentistry
University of California
San Francisco, California

Charles John Palenik, MS, PhD, MBA
Director, Infection Control Research and Services
School of Dentistry
Indiana University
Indianapolis, Indiana

Joseph W. Robertson, DDS
Private Practice
Troy, Michigan

Reviewers

Sharron J. Cook, CDA
Instructor, Dental Assisting
School of Health Sciences
Columbus Technical College
Columbus, Georgia

Heidi Gottfried, BA, CDA
Director and Chairperson
Dental Assisting Program
Gateway Technical College
Kenosha Campus
Kenosha, Wisconsin

Theresa A. Groody, EFDA, CDA, BHS
Expanded Functions Dental Assisting Coordinator
    and Assistant to the Dean of Continuing Studies
Harcum College
Bryn Mawr, Pennsylvania

Preface

The purpose of this book is to provide a steadfast review for the dental assisting student preparing for course review, local or state exams, or for national certification. Three comprehensive tests are included in the same format as the national exam. Tests are divided into the following categories:

- General Chairside (360 questions total/120 questions per test)
- Radiation Health and Safety (300 questions total/100 questions per test)
- Infection Control (300 questions total/100 questions per test)

For added convenience, each question is repeated in the answer key with the rationale for the correct choice so that the results can be checked.

The CD in this book will allow you to test yourself electronically and includes additional practice with the approved Expanded Functions in your state.

ABOUT THE CD

The accompanying CD provides more opportunities to review specific topics. All 960 questions in the book are available electronically. The program lets you choose the topic (General Chairside, Radiation Health and Safety, or Infection Control), and how many questions you want to work through. Questions are randomized from each test, so you will not necessarily see the questions in the same order they appear in the book. Immediate feedback is given after an answer is selected.

The CD also includes questions for a variety of Expanded Functions. Questions can be selected by topic or by state. If you choose the state option, the program will randomize questions for each topic recognized by the state selected.

EXPANDED FUNCTIONS

It should be noted that Expanded Functions (EF) vary by state. The EF questions that are included have not been written for any particular location. We urge all users of this product to be familiar with the current approved EF for their state by contacting the appropriate board of dentistry or other governing agency.

Preparing for a Credentialing Examination—Guidelines for the Candidate

Betty Ladley Finkbeiner

As you open this book you may be asking yourself, "Why am I doing this"? You may think, "I don't need to do this to have a job as a dental assistant". That may be true in some situations but in many regions of the country you need a validated standard of performance in accordance with state dental laws. However, there are many reasons why you should have a professional credential. Anyone who tells you otherwise is not thinking about your professional worth or the importance of such a credential to your patients.

The first and foremost reason for a credential is to practice legally. As a dental assistant you should be familiar with the dental law within the state where you are employed. Many states require documentation of a professional credential to prove your performance in one or more areas of dental assisting. A list of national organizations and contacts for each state's board of examiners is included in the back of this book.

Patients who are in the care of a licensed dentist expect that the dentist will employ qualified personnel. Further they should expect that each of these employees will have completed all the necessary education, and where applicable, secured a professional credential. By obtaining a recognized professional credential in dentistry, you have proven that you have the minimal qualifications to practice the duties that are legally delegable in your state. The credential should be posted where patients can visibly recognize your professional status.

By completing the Dental Assisting National Board (DANB) Certified Dental Assistant (CDA®), Infection Control or Radiography examination, you have validated that you are familiar with the basic concepts of a technical safe practice. This is important to your employer and to the patients who come under your care. Today's patients are concerned with their safety and are aware of potential hazards that exist in health care. You can allay some of those fears if you demonstrate your knowledge in the areas of infection control, radiography, and quality assurance. Further, putting into practice these concepts and the appropriate guidelines from various governing agencies can only serve to protect you, the dental staff, and the patients.

Finally, having a credential that recognizes your knowledge and skills can only serve to increase your self-esteem. For some, this is most important as it shows that you have a documented base of knowledge that is recognized by the dental profession and you have become an important member of the dental health team ... it could also result in a salary increase.

GETTING READY

What is the most important thing a student should do to prepare for an examination?

a. Get a good night's sleep before the examination and eat only a light breakfast.
b. Take two aspirin before entering the examination room to ward off the distraction of a possible headache.
c. Develop an attitude of cautious optimism, that is, "I believe I will pass this examination."
d. Develop a thorough understanding of the body of knowledge and concepts to be covered by the examination.

If you chose "D", you are off to a good start in preparing yourself for any examination, particularly ones like the Dental Assisting National Board or the state board credentialing exams. There is only one way to conquer a well-developed examination—to know the answers to the questions. The "trick" to obtaining good test scores is primarily to retain and apply the knowledge and skills learned in formal course work and in clinical applications. Various ways of helping you develop this strategy will be discussed later.

If you selected "C", you chose an important response but not the "Best" one. It *is* important to go into any examination with a positive attitude and with minimal anxiety, but such an attitude is realistic only if you do have a good command of the subject.

If you chose "A", then perhaps you interpreted the words "prepare for an examination" to mean only those things that should be done on the day before and the day of an exam. But preparation for an examination begins on the day you learn the first vocabulary word or the first concept associated with any area of learning. Exams are just one phase in the total ongoing learning process.

Alternative "B" in the opening example is not a suitable response. It should be obvious that neither aspirin nor any other drug can compensate for knowledge.

Before beginning to study for any type of examination, there are at least three things to do: (1) secure a set of objectives for the area or areas that the examination is designed to evaluate, (2) secure a set of sample questions that are similar to the ones to be used on the examination for which you will be studying, and (3) review the materials in 1 and 2 thoroughly.

LEARNING ABOUT THE EXAMINATION

Whether you are preparing for a national certification examination such as the DANB or a state board or regional credentialing exam you need to be familiar with the material that will be covered. During the application process you will be provided with an outline of the content and rules to follow on examination day. Pay close attention to the content outline and to the number of questions to be asked on each topic. (For information about the DANB examination visit the website at www.danb.org and click on the DANB Exam button on the left.)

If you are taking a state board or regional type examination that includes a clinical component, thoroughly review the list of materials you are to bring. If a patient is part of the clinical component, review the clinical requirements of the patient to ensure that your patient meets the criteria for the exam procedure. You should become familiar with the patient prior to the examination and not be forced to work with an unfamiliar patient. Do not wait until the day before the test to prepare your clinical tray or box since you may find that you do not have access to some material or instrument and may need to buy or borrow some device.

EXAMINATION FORMAT

In addition to knowing the content to be covered, it is important to know that written examinations are usually multiple choice. All questions are apt to be in that format with one best answer for each question.

Many multiple choice questions are written with distracters (responses that are not the answers) that are partially correct or that are correct but are not the best answer.

Some critics of multiple choice tests claim that you can score well on such a test by memorizing facts and learning some tricks to answering such questions. Such criticism is not true for any well developed national or state credentialing examination. The test you take will have been prepared by test specialists. Each test question will have been tried out in regular testing situations with students in classes for dental assistants. You will be taking a great risk if you assume that skillful "guessing" will produce a passing score.

No written examination can test your ability to apply the knowledge or the understanding that you must possess to function as a dental assistant. Some state credentialing exams are apt to include a practical or clinical test, a test in which you will be asked to "demonstrate" what you have learned by doing such things as producing a full crown or intracoronal interim restoration or placing a rubber dam. Any of the clinical tasks, especially expanded functions that you have learned to do, may serve as a "situational" test in which your actual performance is observed and graded. It provides final evidence of whether or not a candidate can "put it all together" and function satisfactorily in a setting that simulates real life in a dental office.

The purpose of any credentialing examination is to determine the extent to which each candidate has mastered the knowledge, concepts, and skills necessary to perform satisfactorily as a dental assistant. No examination, either written or practical, can be long enough to actually cover every concept or skill. Therefore test developers must select questions and practical situations that are typical of the total body of knowledge and skills in dental assisting. As a candidate, you will not know what specific concepts and skills you will be tested on. The only solution is to be well prepared in all aspects of dental assisting.

For written examinations, the multiple choice questions are considered the most versatile. It is a good method for measuring the knowledge of technical vocabulary and specific information that dental assistants must possess. It is also an effective method of measuring your understanding of relationships and interrelationships (which things go together and which do not). It may be used for measuring your application of knowledge to situations that are different from ones you may have previously experienced.

About the only type of cognitive skill that is not measured well by the multiple choice questions is creativity. Although credentialing examinations are designed to find out whether you have mastered the basic fundamental skills of a subject area; they are not designed to discover potential talent for creative innovations.

On any certification, registry, or licensure examination, you will be tested on how well you have acquired and internalized the basic language, concepts, and skills of dental assisting; those things that must become second nature to you as a practicing dental assistant.

STUDYING

The best preparation for a credentialing examination is to be prepared for every dental assisting class that you take. The required textbooks for courses in dental assisting should be studied carefully not only for immediate acquisition of knowledge, but particularly for internalization and retention of that knowledge. Many students find it helpful to highlight key passages in a text so that they can go back and skim those passages easily. This same marking system also works if you have taken online courses and have downloaded lectures. Sometimes the author(s) of a text will emphasize important points for you by paragraph headings or by italicized sentences. Acquisition and retention of important concepts require repetition for most people. Therefore taking the time during an initial reading to make review work easy is time well spent.

Taking good class notes is a very important study skill. Many instructors spend some time making key points and quite a lot of time illustrating these points. Most students are well advised to concentrate on writing down the key points without trying to take notes verbatim. It may be helpful to write down some of your instructor's examples but only if these examples seem necessary to remember the discussion. If the instructor provides outlines or copies of PowerPoint presentations, use a colored marker to highlight important points.

Some students find it difficult to review their own notes after a lecture. It is wise to date the notes, make a heading title on the page, review the notes as soon as possible, and when necessary, recopy the notes for better understanding. If after you have reviewed and edited your notes you have doubts about a concept or basic information, be sure to ask your instructor as soon as possible for clarification.

In addition to identifying the key concepts from text materials, lectures, and notes, it is important to develop a thorough understanding of the dental vocabulary. Every profession has its own vocabulary—not only the technical words that identify important materials, concepts, rules, and ideas, but also the words commonly used to communicate in the profession. Technical vocabulary will be tested in any written or practical exam. In addition, the questions that you will be asked on any credentialing examination will be worded in the day-to-day language of the profession. To progress through the test efficiently, it is essential that you understand quickly and completely each question that you are asked. If you do not understand a question, it will be difficult to answer it correctly.

In addition to the general suggestions for learning and studying throughout your education, there are other options that may be helpful as you review material in preparation for a credentialing examination. Some schools provide review sessions or classes to prepare you. However, if these are not available, one of the most effective steps you can take is to develop cooperative study sessions with one or two friends. Such sessions are best conducted as much like a classroom situation as possible; that is, each person should develop a series of questions to ask the other(s) along with the materials necessary to answer the questions prior to the joint study session. If your colleagues miss any of the questions, you should be prepared to explain the answer to them and vice versa. Teaching the concepts or skill to someone else is one of the best learning techniques to acquire that concept or skill yourself. Consequently, your weakest area is the best one to teach to others. Naturally study sessions such as these are not comparable to a formal class, but they should be conducted in a businesslike fashion. If these study sessions become just a social outing among friends, you may enjoy them, but they will cease to contribute much to your exam preparation.

Regardless of whether you take a formal review class or develop a study session with colleagues, such an experience will likely be very beneficial. A bonus of these sessions is enhanced confidence in your ability to do well in an examination. Nothing builds confidence as much as feeling that you have mastered some area of knowledge or skill so well that you can help others understand it.

FRAME OF MIND

It is wise and prudent to prepare yourself physically for an exam by getting at least 8 hours of sleep and avoiding caffeine. Keep in mind that the test you are taking in dental assisting is to measure your mental abilities not your physical prowess. Studying all night before an examination is not a recommended behavior. Physical fatigue can depress test taking efficiency. The best physical preparation is simply to avoid any major variation from your normal routine.

Preparing for a good mental attitude means that you develop a confidence that you have adequately prepared yourself and that you expect to do well. You may approach an examination with some degree of anxiety, like an athlete who enters a competition. This feeling is not necessarily bad. Research indicates that some test anxiety, as long as it is not severe, may help to produce a positive result.

There is a myth that large numbers of students "clutch" when taking examinations, particularly written examinations. No doubt there are some individuals who have developed psychological blocks to taking tests, but from my teaching experience, I have noted that many (probably most) students who claim that a low test score was caused by an inability to perform well on tests have not developed the requisite knowledge and skills to answer the questions.

Sometimes repeated practice on similar written examinations will be helpful. But if you feel you have a serious test taking problem, it may be necessary to seek some professional counseling to overcome this situation. Some of the following suggestions may help if you have difficulty taking a test.

- Bring all of the necessary admission and testing materials with you.
  - Follow the guidelines provided for you by the testing agency.
- When entering the testing room, choose a seat that will be comfortable for you, unless you are assigned a seat or location.
- Read carefully the printed directions given to you.
- Listen carefully to the verbal directions. Do not assume that because you have taken many examinations that the directions for this one will be the same.
- If the directions are not completely clear to you, ask the examiner in charge of the session to explain exactly what is required.
- Understand completely the mechanics that you are expected to follow during the examination.
- In a written test you will be given multiple choice questions in a booklet and a separate answer sheet.
  - Do not make responses hurriedly or carelessly.
  - Be certain you place your answer on the correct form, correct line and in the space provided.
- On a computer test you will enter your answers on the screen.
  - Be certain that your selection is placed in the correct space provided.
- Be cautious when you correct an answer that your previous answer has either been erased or deleted in either the paper or computer test format.
- Be certain to answer every question.
  - In the computer format, most test formats will indicate that you have not answered specific questions and you can then scroll back to these questions.
  - In a written format, you will need to review your answer sheet for blank spaces to ensure that you have entered an answer for every question.
  - You must arrive at one correct or one "best" answer.
  - If you must, "guess" between two alternatives, eliminate the two or three you know are wrong first.
  - If you can eliminate any responses as incorrect based on your knowledge, you will not be guessing randomly but will be exercising "informed guessing".
- In a clinical examination, you may be expected to select instruments, arrange instruments, and/or perform some other task.
  - Acquaint yourself with the physical facility.
  - If the required procedures are not clear to you, ask for clarification.
- Whether a written or clinical examination, budget your time.
  - Make a quick overview of the number of tasks required in the clinical examination or

the number of questions to be answered in a written examination.

- Think of the pace you will need to follow to allow appropriate amounts of time for each section.
- Remember that some tasks or questions may require more time than others.

• Many test takers find it wise to work all the way through a written exam at a fairly rapid pace by answering first all the questions that they "know" or to which they can work out the answer fairly quickly.

- This method suggests skipping the tough questions the first time through and coming back to them.
- It helps you to build on your own success.
- Success can help to lessen fears or concerns that you may have about the testing situation.
- Sometimes the reading of a question in the middle or toward the end of an examination may trigger your mind with the answer or may provide an important clue for an earlier question.

• Be certain if you skip a question that you take caution in entering the next answer in the appropriate space; double check the question number with the number on the answer sheet or the computer screen.

• Be cautious when reviewing your answer sheet to not make arbitrary changes in your answers.

- Be certain to review the question thoroughly before making an answer change.
- Limited research available suggests the "abler" student tends to increase his or her test scores "a bit" by carefully reviewing items, whereas lower scoring students do not. Go back over questions primarily to check that you have not made some obvious error in such things as reading or marking.

• When taking a clinical examination, many of the same principles apply.

- Proceed cautiously and deliberately, making sure that you understand the task being presented.
- Be certain to review your work to ensure it meets the clinical criteria before indicating you have completed the tasks.

The credentialing examinations available for dental assistants have been designed to allow students to demonstrate knowledge, and show their proficiency in skills essential to begin work as dental professionals. Think of the credentialing examination in dental assisting as an opportunity to demonstrate professional competency in your chosen field. Preparation for such an exam is preparation for your chosen profession.

Acknowledgments

The publisher wishes to thank Betty Ladley Finkbeiner for her expertise and leadership in this project. Her work ethic and many insights were an inspiration to us all.

Contents

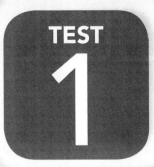

TEST 1

General Chairside, Radiation Health and Safety, and Infection Control

General Chairside

Directions: Select the response that best answers each of the following questions. Only one response is correct.

1. The position of the body standing erect with the feet together and the arms hanging at the sides with the palms facing forward is referred to as the:
   a. resting position
   b. anatomic position
   c. supine position
   d. postural position

2. In the illustration shown, Dr. Curtis was assisted by Debbie May Ross to complete operative treatment for this patient. What required data are missing from the chart?
   a. file number or "NA" if not used, date of the appointment, dentist's initials
   b. time of the appointment, amount of cavity medication used, dentist's initials
   c. type of dental material, amount of cavity medication used, assistant's initials
   d. file number or "NA" if not used, assistant's initials

PROGRESS NOTES

Name _Whitworth, Kimberly_____ Birth date _10/27/69_ File #_____ Page___1___

| _11/19/00_ | _19MD 2C Carbo., Life, A   JWC_ |

3. The examination technique in which the examiner uses his or her fingers and hands to feel for size, texture, and consistency of hard and soft tissue is called:
   a. detection
   b. palpation
   c. probing
   d. extraoral examination

4. Which type of consent is given when a patient enters a dentist's office?
   a. informed consent
   b. implied consent
   c. implied consent for minors
   d. informed refusal

5. Consent is:
   a. an involuntary act
   b. voluntary acceptance or agreement to what is planned or done by another person
   c. only necessary for surgical procedures
   d. something that any person over 21 may give for another's treatment

6. A patient's chart that denotes abnormally small jaws would indicate:
   a. micrognathia
   b. macrodontia
   c. macrognathia
   d. anodontia

7. The tooth-numbering system that begins with the maxillary right third molar as tooth No. 1 and ends with the mandibular right third molar as tooth No. 32 is the:
   a. Universal System
   b. Palmer Notation System
   c. Fédération Dentaire Internationale System
   d. Bracket Numbering System

8. An abbreviation used in the progress notes or chart to indicate a mesioocclusobuccal restoration would be:
   a. BuOcM
   b. BOM
   c. MOD
   d. MOB

9. A hereditary abnormality in which there are defects in the enamel formation is:
   a. germination
   b. fusion
   c. ankylosis
   d. amelogenesis imperfecta

10. Any tooth that remains unerupted in the jaw beyond the time at which it should normally erupt is referred to as being:
   a. abraded
   b. impacted
   c. ankylosed
   d. fused

11. An oral habit consisting of involuntary gnashing, grinding, and clenching of the teeth is:
   a. bulimia
   b. bruxism
   c. attrition
   d. abrasion

12. A horizontal or transverse plane divides the body into:
   a. superior and inferior portions
   b. dorsal and ventral portions
   c. anterior and posterior portions
   d. medial and lateral portions

13. The cells associated with bone formation are known as:
   a. osteoclasts
   b. cancellous cells
   c. cortical cells
   d. osteoblasts

14. Which of the following teeth generally have two roots?
   a. maxillary first molars
   b. mandibular first molars
   c. maxillary second premolars
   d. maxillary central incisors

15. Which of the following is *not* a function of the paranasal sinuses?
   a. lighten the skull
   b. provide resonance
   c. aid in digestion
   d. warm respired air

16. How many teeth are in the arch of a deciduous dentition?
   a. 10
   b. 20
   c. 32
   d. 52

17. The tooth that has two roots and five cusps of which three are on the buccal and two are on the lingual would be a:
   a. maxillary first molar
   b. maxillary first premolar
   c. mandibular first molar
   d. mandibular second molar

18. A 10-year-old patient would likely have which of the following teeth?
   a. permanent mandibular central and lateral incisors, primary second molars, permanent mandibular canines, permanent first molars
   b. permanent mandibular central and lateral incisors, permanent first and second premolars, primary second molars, permanent first molars
   c. primary mandibular central and lateral incisors, primary second molars, permanent canines, permanent first molars
   d. permanent mandibular canines, primary central and lateral incisors, primary second molars, permanent first molars

19. What is the average range of the body's oral resting temperature?
   a. 93.5° F to 99.5° F
   b. 95° F to 99.5° F
   c. 96.5° F to 100° F
   d. 97.6° F to 99° F

20. The most common site for taking a patient's pulse in the dental office is the:
   a. brachial artery
   b. carotid artery
   c. radial artery
   d. femoral artery

21. The primary step in preventing a medical emergency is to be certain the patient has _____ before treatment is begun.
    a. eaten
    b. taken all assigned medications
    c. completed and updated their medical history
    d. signed a consent form

22. Which of the following is each member of the dental team *not* required to have the knowledge and skills to perform prior to handling an emergency in the dental office?
    a. current credentials to perform basic life support or cardiopulmonary resuscitation (CPR)
    b. current certification to administer all cardiac medications
    c. current credentials to perform the Heimlich maneuver
    d. ability to obtain and record vital signs

23. The ABCDs of basic life support stand for:
    a. access, breath, care, and dial
    b. airway, breathing, circulation, and dial
    c. airway, breathing, circulation, and defibrillation
    d. assess, breath, care, and dial

24. The most frequently used substance in a medical emergency is:
    a. glucose
    b. oxygen
    c. epinephrine
    d. ammonia inhalant

25. The dental assistant's responsibility in an emergency situation is:
    a. to recognize the symptoms and signs of a significant medical complaint
    b. to provide appropriate support in implementing emergency procedures
    c. to identify a specific condition or emergency situation
    d. both a and b

26. _____, which is precipitated by stress and anxiety, may manifest in rapid, shallow breathing; lightheadedness; rapid heartbeat; and a panic-stricken appearance and is treated by having the patient breathe into a paper bag or cupped hands.
    a. Asthma attack
    b. Hyperventilation
    c. Allergic reaction
    d. Angina

27. The list of emergency telephone numbers posted next to each telephone throughout the office should include all *except* _____.
    a. police and firefighters
    b. nearest hospital, physicians, and oral surgeons
    c. patient emergency numbers
    d. EMS system

28. To ensure that a medical emergency is observed immediately, it is important for the dental assistant to:
    a. check the patient's pulse periodically during treatment
    b. check the patient's blood pressure periodically during treatment
    c. be alert to continuously observe the patient to note any potential problems
    d. ask the patient periodically how he or she feels

29. The three characteristics noted in the patient record when measuring respirations are:
a. rate, rhythm, and flow
b. rate, rhythm, and depth
c. volume, flow, and rate
d. volume, flow, and depth

Use the following chart to answer questions 30 and 31.

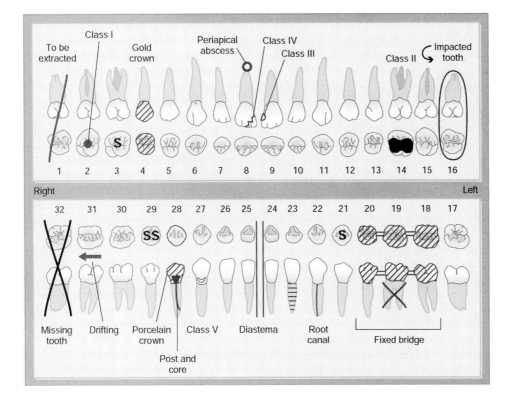

30. The symbol on tooth No. 3 indicates that this tooth:
a. has a sealant placed
b. has a stainless steel crown
c. needs to have a sealant
d. has occlusal staining

31. The symbols on teeth Nos. 18 through 20 indicate that:
a. No. 19 is a full gold crown
b. No. 19 is missing and a bridge is present
c. Nos. 18 and 20 are missing
d. Nos. 18 and 20 are pontics

32. Based on the chart given here, how many permanent teeth are present on the mandible?
   a. 6
   b. 10
   c. 12
   d. 14

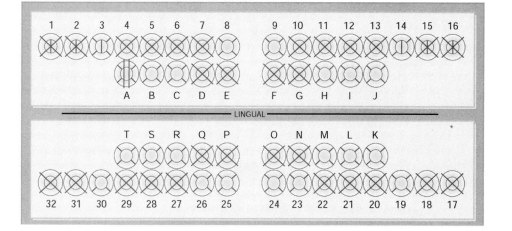

33. When a patient's pulse is being taken, his or her arm should be:
   a. well supported and above his or her shoulder
   b. hanging loosely between his or her knees
   c. unsupported and extended below the waist
   d. well supported, extended and positioned at the same level or lower than the heart

34. Motion economy is the concept that encourages the dental health care worker to:
   a. increase the number and length of motions at chairside
   b. decrease the number and length of motions at chairside
   c. use quick motions to save energy
   d. use slow deliberate motions that exercise the arm to reduce stress

35. Which of the following devices might *not* be found on a prophylaxis tray?
   a. cotton-tipped applicator
   b. gauze sponge
   c. straight fissure plain cut bur
   d. polishing cup

36. Which of the following devices would be a choice for checking a patient's occlusion during an oral prophylaxis?
   a. cotton-tipped applicator
   b. gauze sponge
   c. articulating paper
   d. straight fissure cross cut bur

37. Which of the following should be done if the patient has thick, heavy saliva that adheres to the prophylaxis cup during the polishing procedure?
 a. place a saliva ejector in the mouth instead of using the HVE tip
 b. keep the HVE tip as close as possible to the polishing cup
 c. do not polish the teeth
 d. have the patient rinse out in the sink after all the polishing is done

38. What prosthetic device replaces missing teeth by metal framework and artificial teeth?
 a. maxillary denture
 b. mandibular partial denture
 c. bridge
 d. restoration

39. The portion of a bridge that replaces the missing tooth is called a(n):
 a. denture
 b. abutment
 c. pontic
 d. root

40. Which of the following instruments would be used to measure the depth of the gingival sulcus?
 a. periodontal probe
 b. cowhorn explorer
 c. right angle explorer
 d. shepherd's hook

41. Which of the following instruments is used to scale deep periodontal pockets or furcation areas?
 a. curette scaler
 b. Gracey scaler
 c. straight sickle scaler
 d. modified sickle scaler

42. The HVE system is used:
 a. to remove liquids slowly
 b. to remove large volumes of fluid and debris from the mouth
 c. primarily during surgical procedures
 d. most commonly during a prophylaxis

43. Which of the following instruments can be used to invert the rubber dam?
 a. explorer
 b. spoon excavator
 c. Svedopter
 d. floss

44. If treatment is to be performed on tooth No. 13, which of the following is true about clamp placement?
 a. The clamp is placed on No. 14, and Nos. 14 through 11 are isolated.
 b. The clamp is placed on No. 15, and Nos. 15 through 12 are isolated.
 c. The clamp is placed on No. 13, and Nos. 14 through 11 are isolated.
 d. The clamp is placed on No. 12, and Nos. 12 through 15 are isolated.

45. You are assisting a right-handed operator in a procedure performed on the patient's left side. The HVE tip and A/W syringe are being used. The operator signals for a transfer. You must:
    a. return the A/W to the dental unit, hold onto the HVE, and pick up the new instrument to be transferred
    b. transfer the A/W syringe to the right hand, retain the HVE tip in the right hand, and pick up the new instrument to be transferred
    c. lay both the HVE and A/W syringe across your lap, and pick up the new instrument to be transferred
    d. give a signal to the dentist/operator that you are unable to make the transfer at this time

46. Which of the following is *not* a correct statement for seating the operating team?
    a. The operator's thighs are parallel to the floor.
    b. The assistant's thighs are parallel to the floor.
    c. The operator is always seated at the 12 o'clock position.
    d. The mobile cart is placed close to the patient chair.

47. When placing the amalgam into the preparation for a 31DO restoration, the first increment should be placed into the:
    a. distoocclusal region
    b. proximal box
    c. mesioocclusal region
    d. midocclusal region

48. Which of the following instruments would be used to grasp tissue or bone fragments during a surgical procedure?
    a. hemostat
    b. locking endodontic pliers
    c. periosteal elevator
    d. rongeur forceps

49. Which of the following is the common choice in providing for retention in a cavity preparation?
    a. No. 34 high speed
    b. No. 57 low speed
    c. No. 2, 3, or 6 low speed
    d. No. ½ on low or high speed

50. Which of these would *not* be a form of matrix for an anterior esthetic restoration?
    a. celluloid strip
    b. celluloid crown
    c. universal metal matrix band
    d. Class V composite matrix

51. When placing a composite restoration on the buccal cervical of tooth No. 30, which is the choice of matrix?
    a. universal circumferential metal matrix
    b. Class V composite matrix
    c. celluloid strip
    d. celluloid crown

52. The most common form of anesthesia used in operative dentistry is:
   a. local
   b. conscious sedation
   c. inhalation
   d. general

53. For dental professionals, the safest allowable amount of N_2O is _____ parts per million.
   a. 50
   b. 75
   c. 100
   d. 1000

54. Which of the following medical conditions is *not* a contraindication to using a vasoconstrictor in the local anesthesia during operative treatment?
   a. recent heart attack
   b. uncontrolled heart failure
   c. recent coronary artery bypass surgery
   d. diabetes

55. _____ is frequently used on the mandibular teeth and is injected near a major nerve that anesthetizes the entire area served by that nerve branch.
   a. Block anesthesia
   b. Infiltration anesthesia
   c. Innervation anesthesia
   d. Induction anesthesia

56. Nitrous oxide oxygen administration always begins and ends with:
   a. the patient deep breathing
   b. the patient breathing 100% oxygen
   c. taking the patient's blood pressure and temperature
   d. providing a glass of water or other cold beverage

57. Which of the following is *not* a form of a retention aid for a crown when the tooth is extensively decayed, is fractured, or has had endodontic treatment?
   a. resin-bonded bracket
   b. core buildup
   c. retention pins
   d. post and core

58. The tray setup in the photograph is used to:
    a. place separators
    b. fit and cement orthodontic bands
    c. directly bond orthodontic bands
    d. place and remove ligature ties

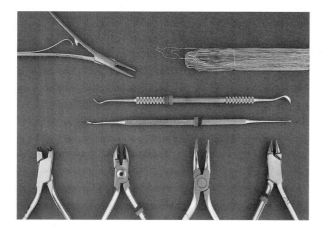

59. To control swelling after a surgical procedure, the patient should be instructed to:
    a. place a cold pack in a cycle of 20 minutes on and 20 minutes off for the first 24 hours
    b. place a cold pack in a cycle of 60 minutes on and 60 minutes off for the first 12 hours
    c. place a cold pack in a cycle of 20 minutes on and 20 minutes off for the first 12 hours, then apply heat in the same form for the next 12 hours
    d. place a heat pack in a cycle of 20 minutes on and 20 minutes off for the first 24 hours

60. A painful condition that can occur after a surgical extraction is inflammation known as _____, also known as _____.
    a. periodontitis, lost granulation tissue
    b. alveolitis, dry socket
    c. hemostasis, dry socket
    d. hemostasis, granulation tissue

61. It may take _____ to complete a dental implant procedure.
    a. 1 month
    b. 6 to 8 weeks
    c. 3 to 9 months
    d. 1 year

62. A metal frame that is placed under the periosteum and on top of the bone is called a(n):
    a. endosteal implant
    b. subperiosteal implant
    c. transosteal implant
    d. triseptal implant

63. The natural rubber material used to obturate the pulp canal after treatment is completed is called:
    a. silver point
    b. gutta-percha
    c. glass ionomer
    d. endodontic filler

64. In this photograph, which instrument is a barbed broach?

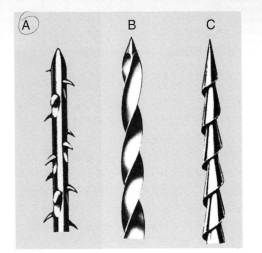

A   B   C

65. A common solution used for irrigation during the debridement procedure in endodontic treatment is:
   a. sodium chloride
   b. sterile saline solution
   c. sodium hypochlorite
   d. sterile water

66. The incisional periodontal surgical procedure that does not remove tissues but pushes away the underlying tooth roots and alveolar bone is known as:
   a. gingivectomy
   b. gingivoplasty
   c. flap surgery
   d. apicoectomy

67. Which of the following does *not* contribute to periodontal disease?
   a. pathologic migration
   b. bruxism
   c. mobility
   d. tooth eruption time

68. The _____ is an instrument that resembles a large spoon and is used to debride the interior of the socket to remove diseased tissue and abscesses.
   a. root tip elevator
   b. rongeur
   c. surgical curette
   d. hemostat

69. From the instruments shown here, select the curette.

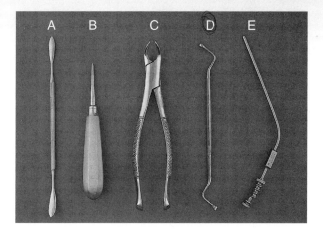

70. Coronal polishing is a technique used for all of the following purposes *except* _____.
   a. to remove plaque and stains from coronal surfaces of the teeth
   b. before placement of dental sealants and orthodontic bands
   c. to remove calculus from subgingival surfaces
   d. before placement of the dental dam and before acid etching

71. Exogenous stains are caused by an environmental source and are classified into subdivisions, including which of the following?
   a. endogenous
   b. extrinsic stains
   c. intrinsic stains
   d. a and c
   e. b and c

72. For which purpose is disclosing solution *not* used?
   a. identifying areas of plaque
   b. desensitizing cervical surfaces
   c. showing intrinsic stain
   d. evaluating the effectiveness of polishing

73. The first step in placing dental sealants is to _____ the surface.
   a. etch
   b. isolate
   c. clean
   d. prime

74. Enamel that has been etched has the appearance of being:
   a. chalky
   b. shiny
   c. wet
   d. slightly brown

75. According to Black's classification of cavities, the type of decay diagnosed on the incisal edge of anterior teeth and the cusp tips of posterior teeth is _____.
   a. Class VI
   b. Class IV
   c. Class II
   d. Class V

76. The isolation of multiple anterior teeth requires the dental dam be placed _____.
   a. only on the one tooth being restored
   b. on the tooth being restored and on one tooth distal on each side
   c. from premolar to premolar
   d. from first molar to first molar

77. When one or more teeth are missing from the same quadrant, a permanent _____ would most commonly be recommended by the dentist.
   a. partial denture
   b. full denture
   c. full crowns
   d. fixed bridge

78. Gingival retraction cord is placed _____ the crown preparation is completed and is removed _____ the final impression is taken.
   a. after, after
   b. before, before
   c. before, after
   d. after, before

79. A _____ is an orthodontic _____ that is a custom appliance made of rubber or pliable acrylic that fits over the patient's dentition after orthodontic treatment.
   a. Harding retainer, arch wire
   b. Hawley retainer, fixed appliance
   c. headgear, positioner
   d. Hawley retainer, positioner

80. This tray set-up is for:
  a. band removal
  b. placing and removing elastometric ties
  c. placing separators
  d. placing arch wires

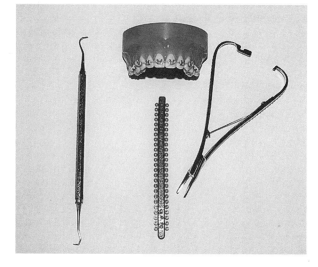

81. Instrument "A" in the photograph is used to:
  a. insert the orthodontic band
  b. force the band down onto the middle third of the tooth
  c. aid in forcing the cement out of the band
  d. open the buccal tube

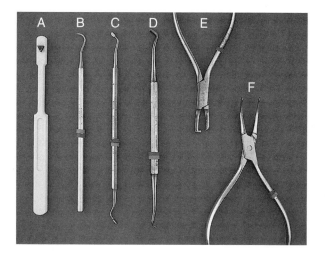

82. A(n) _____ is used to provide interproximal space for inserting an orthodontic band.
  a. arch wire
  b. bracket
  c. separator
  d. band

83. _____, also known as *tongue tied*, results in a short lingual frenum.
    a. Macrodontia
    b. Microdontia
    c. Ankyloglossia
    d. Anodontia

84. _____ is a condition in which an inflammation is uncontrolled within a localized area and spreads throughout the soft tissue and organ.
    a. Angular cheilitis
    b. Cellulitis
    c. Glossitis
    d. Oral cancer

85. _____ is a superficial infection caused by a yeast-like fungus.
    a. Leukoplakia
    b. Lichen planus
    c. Candidiasis
    d. Aphthous ulcer

86. Which instrument would be used to remove the right mandibular first molar?

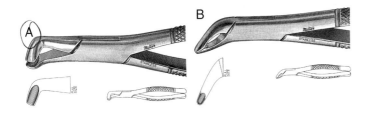

87. Which instrument would be used to remove the right maxillary second molar?

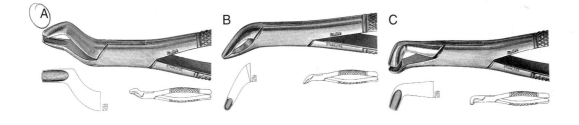

88. Using Black's classification of cavities, a lesion on the cervical third of a tooth is considered a Class _____ restoration or cavity.
    a. I
    b. II
    c. III
    d. V

89. Which of the following teeth are not succedaneous?
    a. permanent central incisors
    b. permanent canines
    c. permanent first molars
    d. permanent premolars

90. The automatic external defibrillator (AED) is used for all *except* _____.
    a. to reestablish the proper heart rhythm
    b. to automatically perform CPR for 15 minutes
    c. to shock the heart
    d. to monitor the patient's heart rhythm

91. Which of the following is *not* a characteristic that allows dental materials to withstand the oral environment?
    a. mechanical properties and electrical properties
    b. corrosive properties and thermal properties
    c. solubility and application properties
    d. trituration and amalgamation properties

92. A dental restorative material that is applied to a tooth or teeth while the material is pliable and can be adapted, carved, and finished is classified as:
    a. direct restorations
    b. indirect restorations
    c. crowns, bridges, or onlays
    d. implants

93. Which of these would have the least dimensional stability?
    a. silicone
    b. polysiloxane
    c. alginate hydrocolloid
    d. agar hydrocolloid

94. The conventional or traditional composites, which contain the largest filler particles and provide the greatest strength, are known as:
    a. microfilled composites
    b. hybrid composites
    c. midfilled composites
    d. macrofilled composites

95. If a light bodied impression catalyst is mixed with a heavy bodied impression base, the resultant mix might:
    a. be discolored
    b. set improperly
    c. polymerize immediately
    d. not mix

96. Addition of cold water to an alginate mix will cause the setting time to be:
    a. increased
    b. decreased

97. Select two terms that describe the purpose and consistency of a dental cement used for the final seating of a porcelain fused-to-metal crown.
  a. base and secondary consistency
  b. cementation and secondary consistency
  c. base and primary consistency
  d. cementation and primary consistency

98. Noble metals used in indirect restorations include all *except* _____.
  a. gold and palladium
  b. gold and platinum
  c. gold and mercury
  d. palladium and platinum

99. Which of the following statements is *not* true about the use of calcium hydroxide as a frequently selected cavity liner?
  a. It protects the pulp from chemical irritation through its sealing abilities.
  b. It stimulates the production of reparative or secondary dentin.
  c. It is the most cost-effective liner for use under all types of restorations.
  d. It is compatible with all types of restorative materials.

100. The advantage of using a glass ionomer restorative material is:
  a. it releases an obtundant
  b. it releases fluoride after its final setting
  c. it does not need to be cured
  d. it has the strongest compressive strength of any restorative material

101. A custom tray is constructed to fit the mouth of a specific patient and is used to _____, _____, and _____.
  a. save money, reduce chair time, reduce patient discomfort
  b. adapt to the patient's mouth, fit around any anomalies, reduce the amount of impression material needed
  c. adapt to the patient's mouth, aid the laboratory technician, provide for a better restoration
  d. reduce patient cost, reduce chair time, reduce patient discomfort

102. Which form of gypsum product is commonly used for making diagnostic models?
  a. plaster
  b. dental stone
  c. high-strength stone
  d. impression plaster

103. When taking impressions, the next step after seating the patient and placing the patient napkin is to:
  a. assemble the materials needed
  b. mix the impression material
  c. explain the procedure to the patient
  d. record treatment on the chart

104. Prior to handing a record to the administrative assistant after treating a patient, the clinical assistant should:
  a. retain the gloves used during the procedure so as not to delay the patient's checkout at the business office
  b. remove clinical gloves and put on polynitrile gloves
  c. remove the contaminated gloves and wash hands
  d. place polynitrile gloves over the clinical gloves to prevent cross contamination outside the treatment room

105. The information in a registration form should include all *except* _____.
    a. name, address, and phone number of person responsible for the account
    b. place of employment of the responsible party
    c. information concerning the patient's coverage under an insurance plan
    d. age of all dependents

106. Financial arrangements for treatment should *not* be made:
    a. in private
    b. before treatment begins
    c. after treatment is completed
    d. by the business assistant

107. _____ is the amount the dental assistant takes home after all the deductions are made.
    a. Gross pay
    b. Net pay
    c. Withholding
    d. FICA

108. _____ is another name for the Social Security funds deducted from an employee's pay.
    a. Withholding
    b. FICA
    c. Federal tax
    d. Gross wage

109. Which of these is an expendable item used in the dental office?
    a. hemostat
    b. instrument cassette
    c. latex gloves
    d. computer software

110. Which is a capital item in a dental office?
    a. hemostat
    b. cotton rolls
    c. x-ray unit
    d. computer software

111. Oxygen should be stored:
    a. horizontally in a cool place
    b. vertically and secured
    c. horizontally in a warm place
    d. outside the office

112. An office system that tracks patients' follow-up visits for an oral prophylaxis is a(n):
    a. screening system
    b. on-call record
    c. recall system
    d. tickler file

113. Which of the following statements should be reworded on a patient's record to avoid litigation?
    a. The patient experienced difficulty in holding the impression in the mouth.
    b. The patient was not used to the new laser system used for the procedure.
    c. This patient was a real problem and disrupted our entire day.
    d. The patient apologized for being unable to hold the impression long enough.

114. What are the consequences of using a nickname or an incorrect name when filing an insurance claim form?
    a. no payment will ever be made
    b. processing of the form will be delayed
    c. there are no consequences
    d. there will be an underpayment

115. An administrative assistant records information the dentist dictates for a patient's clinical record after the treatment is complete. Later, litigation is taken against the dentist in the practice for treatment that was rendered. The administrative assistant is asked to testify. Which of the following statements is *true*?
    a. The administrative assistant is an expert witness.
    b. The administrative assistant is an eyewitness.
    c. The administrative assistant can only testify to what he or she was told to write in the record.
    d. The administrative assistant should refuse to testify.

116. When speaking to a patient on the telephone, which is the most courteous action?
    a. hang up as soon as possible
    b. wait for the patient to hang up and then hang up
    c. tell the patient when you are going to hang up
    d. close the conversation and hang up quickly so the patient does not continue the conversation

117. The leading cause of tooth loss in adults is:
    a. dental caries
    b. aging
    c. periodontal disease
    d. lack of home care

118. The first step in patient education is to:
    a. instruct the patient how to remove plaque
    b. select home care aids
    c. listen carefully to the patient
    d. reinforce home care

119. The MyPyramid, formerly known as the Food Guide Pyramid, is an outline of what to eat each day. The largest section on the pyramid is in what food group?
    a. dairy
    b. meat
    c. grains
    d. vegetables

120. Which of the following statements is *false* regarding carbohydrates?
    a. They provide energy.
    b. They are found in grains, fruits, and vegetables.
    c. They provide vitamins.
    d. Complex carbohydrates are the major source for dental caries.

Radiation Health and Safety

Directions: Select the response that best answers each of the following questions. Only one response is correct.

1. Radiographs are used in an oral diagnosis to detect all of the following *except* _____.
   a. periodontal disease
   b. defective restorations
   c. malocclusion
   d. pathologic conditions

2. In the radiograph below, what is the lesion at the apex of the mandibular central incisor?
   a. periapical cyst
   b. periodontal abscess
   c. osseous stone
   d. condensing osteitis

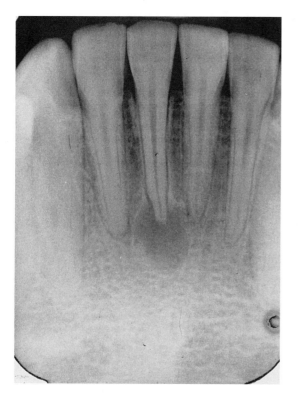

3. Commercially available barrier envelopes:
   a. minimize contamination before exposure of the film
   b. minimize contamination after exposure of the film
   c. are made of a material that blocks the passage of photons
   d. are made of a material that blocks the passage of electrons

4. Preparation of supplies and equipment involves sterilizing which of the following items?
   a. film
   b. film-holding device
   c. lead apron
   d. PID

5. Exposed films should _____ dried and then placed in a _____ for transport to the darkroom for processing.
   a. not be, gloved hand
   b. be, gloved hand
   c. not be, disposable container
   d. be, disposable container

6. When handling film with barrier envelopes, the barrier envelopes are opened with _____ hands and the films unwrapped with _____ hands.
   a. gloved, gloved
   b. gloved, nongloved
   c. nongloved, gloved
   d. nongloved, nongloved

7. Root fractures occur most often in the _____ region.
   a. maxillary central incisors
   b. mandibular central incisors
   c. maxillary molars
   d. mandibular molars

8. The _____ radiograph is the film of choice for the evaluation of mandibular fractures.
   a. occlusal
   b. periapical
   c. bitewing
   d. panoramic

9. Overlapped interproximal contacts result from:
   a. incorrect vertical angulation
   b. incorrect horizontal angulation
   c. film placement
   d. processing errors

10. The quality of the x-ray photos is determined by the:
   a. kilovoltage
   b. collimation
   c. milliamperage
   d. HVL factor

11. When using the bisecting method the object-film distance is kept to a _____.
   a. maximum
   b. minimum

12. The advantage of double-emulsion intraoral films over the old single emulsion films is:
   a. more flexibility
   b. faster developing time
   c. less radiation exposure to patients
   d. increased darkroom illumination

13. Taking the film to be duplicated out of the mounts:
   a. improves the contrast of the duplicates
   b. makes processing easier
   c. improves the detail of the duplicates
   d. prolongs the life of the duplicating device

14. A tissue that lies within the primary dental beam and receives a lot of secondary radiation is the _____.
   a. tongue
   b. cornea
   c. thyroid
   d. inner ear

15. Reticulation of the emulsion is usually the result of:
   a. excessive drying
   b. improper fixing
   c. inadequate rinsing
   d. a sudden change in temperature between the developer solution and the water bath

16. All of the following affect the life of processing solutions *except* _____.
   a. number of films processed
   b. size of films processed
   c. age of the solutions
   d. type of safelight

17. If the manual developing time is 5 minutes, then the fixing time should be _____.
   a. 2.5 minutes
   b. 5 minutes
   c. 8 minutes
   d. 10 minutes

18. The protective coating on the emulsion is softened by the _____ and hardened by the _____.
   a. fixer, developer
   b. developer, water rinse
   c. developer, fixer
   d. fixer, water rinse

19. Barrier pack films should be used for:
   a. all patients
   b. patients with a positive medical history
   c. patients who are bleeding
   d. patients with contaminated saliva

20. Dark films can be caused by:
   a. increased focal-film distance
   b. increased object-film distance
   c. overexposure
   d. underdevelopment

21. In a full mouth survey:
    a. periapical films of edentulous areas are not taken
    b. bitewing films of edentulous areas are taken
    c. periapical films of edentulous areas are always taken
    d. opposing teeth for bitewings are not necessary

22. An overexposed film will appear similar to an _____ film.
    a. overdeveloped
    b. underdeveloped

23. Reversing the film to the x-ray beam will cause a _____.
    a. darkened film
    b. geometric pattern
    c. clear film
    d. black film

24. When using the bisecting techniques, the imaginary angle that is bisected is formed between the long axis of the tooth and the:
    a. long axis of the PID
    b. horizontal axis of the film
    c. long axis of the film
    d. horizontal axis of the tube head

25. The technique or concept that provides for the orientation of structures seen in two radiographs exposed at different angles to determine the buccal-lingual relationship of an object is referred to as the _____.
    a. Compton electron rule
    b. Bremsstrahlung
    c. buccal object rule
    d. cone-beam technology

26. In the bisecting technique the tooth-film distance is:
    a. maximal
    b. minimum
    c. not important
    d. decreased by 0.5 inch

27. All bitewings are taken using the:
    a. paralleling technique
    b. bisecting technique
    c. protrusive relation
    d. visual focal technique

28. The marked prominence that appears on a maxillary molar periapical film as a triangular radiopacity superimposed over, or inferior to, the maxillary tuberosity region is:
    a. the hard palate
    b. a fracture line
    c. the coronoid process
    d. the maxillary sinus

29. The main disadvantage of panoramic films is:
   a. increased patient exposure
   b. loss of definition and detail
   c. lack of contrast
   d. possible patient movement

30. Which of the following methods is best for taking a radiograph of an impacted third molar on the mandible?
   a. posterior anterior
   b. lateral oblique
   c. lateral skull
   d. posterior anterior of the sinuses

31. Cassettes with intensifying screens are used in extraoral radiography to _____.
   a. decrease patient exposure
   b. decrease patient chair time
   c. decrease processing time
   d. eliminate processing time

32. A conventional panoramic projection will show both the right and left joints in the:
   a. lateral plane
   b. axial plane
   c. cross-sectional plane
   d. frontal plane

33. One advantage of the storage phosphor technique is that the sensor is:
   a. larger
   b. smaller
   c. slightly more flexible
   d. more sensitive to radiation

34. The definition seen on a digital image compared with film is:
   a. the same
   b. better
   c. slightly less
   d. exaggerated

35. Three types of direct sensors are _____, _____, and _____.
   a. CMOS, MCD, CID
   b. XCP, CMOS, CUD
   c. CMOS, CCD, CID
   d. XCP, CCD, CID

36. The main disadvantage of a metal rubber dam holder in endodontics is:
   a. it is bendable
   b. it is easier to use
   c. it is harder to remove
   d. its image will be superimposed on the film

37. On intraoral radiographs, when the patient's right is on your left, this is called _____ mounting.
   a. labial
   b. neutral
   c. cross
   d. lingual

38. On a routine full mouth survey, it is not possible to see the_____ foramen.
   a. mental
   b. incisive
   c. lingual
   d. mandibular

39. It is difficult radiographically to differentiate dentin from:
   a. bone
   b. enamel
   c. cementum
   d. pulp

40. Most lesions appear _____ on processed radiographs.
   a. radiopaque
   b. radiolucent
   c. geometric
   d. poorly defined

41. Caries that radiographically involve the dentin are classified as _____.
   a. early
   b. late
   c. incipient
   d. advanced

42. An example of caries that is almost never seen on a radiograph is _____.
   a. incisal
   b. interproximal
   c. lingual
   d. incipient

43. Temporary acrylic crowns appear _____ on radiographs.
   a. radiolucent
   b. radiopaque

44. Gold crowns appear _____ on radiographs.
   a. radiolucent
   b. radiopaque

45. Cement bases under restorations appear _____ on a radiograph.
   a. radiolucent
   b. radiopaque

46. Bitewing projections cannot be used to detect:
   a. caries
   b. bone levels
   c. root fractures
   d. restorations

47. High pulp horns on teeth are usually associated with _____.
   a. elderly patients
   b. young patients
   c. teenagers
   d. male children

48. Fractures of the mandible will appear:
   a. not on a periapical film
   b. as a radiopaque line
   c. as a radiolucent line
   d. only if observed within the first 24 hours

49. Implants will appear _____ on radiographs.
   a. radiolucent
   b. radiopaque

50. To obtain the best definition of a suspected residual root tip, a _____ projection should be used.
   a. bitewing
   b. periapical
   c. panoramic
   d. tomograph

51. A malignant tumor of bone will appear _____ on radiographs.
   a. radiolucent
   b. radiopaque

52. An enlarged and bulbous, or club shaped, root is usually a sign of _____.
   a. pathology
   b. concrescence
   c. hypercementosis
   d. cemental dysplasia

53. Treating a patient without proper radiographs is a breach of the _____.
   a. law of ALARA
   b. inverse square law
   c. MPD
   d. standard of care

54. Original radiographs should always be kept in the:
   a. dental office
   b. patient's possession
   c. insurance office
   d. off-site security office

55. The concept that the dental practitioner should expose the patient to the least amount of radiation exposure within the dental office without excessive cost refers to the _____.
   a. Heinz principle
   b. ALARA principle
   c. dental insurance regulations
   d. OSHA regulations

56. The film below illustrates:
   a. bent film with a thin radiolucent line
   b. film crease with a thin radiopaque line
   c. bent film with distortion
   d. film crease with a thin radiolucent line

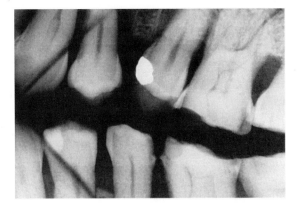

57. When a clear (unexposed) area appears on the film:
   a. the PID was not directed at the center of the film
   b. the horizontal angulation was incorrect
   c. the kVp setting was incorrect
   d. the mA setting was incorrect

58. When overlapped contacts appear on the film:
   a. the vertical angulation was incorrect
   b. the central ray was not directed through the interproximal spaces
   c. the film was bent
   d. the film was improperly placed

Review the image below to answer questions 59 and 60.

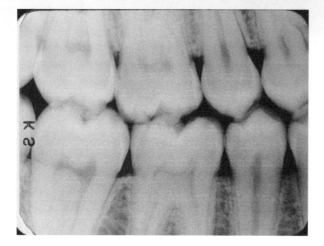

59. What is the problem with the molar bitewing?
  a. the third molar regions are not visible on the film
  b. the premolars are not all on the film
  c. the apices do not appear
  d. the second premolar is not in the middle of the film

60. By changing the _____, the clinical value of this film could be improved.
  a. vertical angulation
  b. horizontal angulation
  c. film placement
  d. film size

61. _____ is the error in the film below.
  a. Vertical angulation
  b. Horizontal angulation
  c. Film placement
  d. Film size

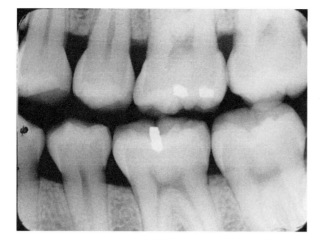

62. The error in the radiograph below is:
   a. incorrect film placement
   b. cone cutting
   c. increased kVp
   d. decreased mA

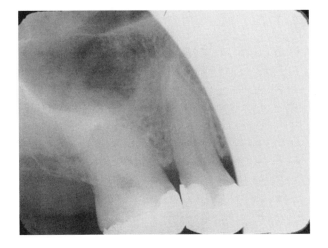

63. The error in the radiograph below is:
   a. incorrect film placement
   b. cone cutting
   c. increased kVp
   d. decreased mA

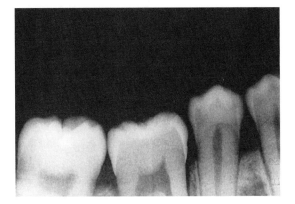

64. The error in the radiograph below is:
   a. vertical angulation
   b. horizontal angulation
   c. film placement
   d. film size

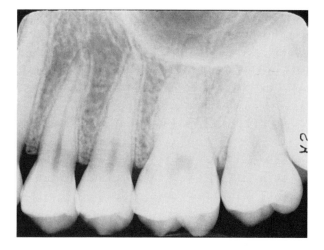

Review the image below to answer questions 65 and 66.

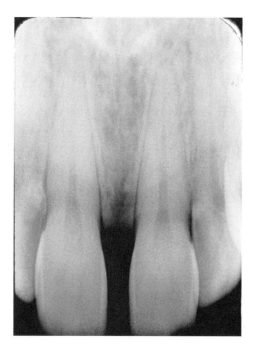

65. The error in this radiograph is:
   a. foreshortening
   b. elongation
   c. cone cutting
   d. bent film

66. The error in this radiograph can be corrected by changing the:
   a. vertical angulation
   b. horizontal angulation
   c. film placement
   d. film size

Review the image below to answer questions 67 and 68.

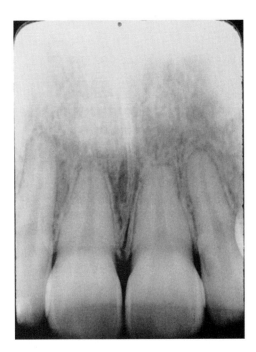

67. The error in this radiograph is:
   a. foreshortening
   b. elongation
   c. cone cutting
   d. bent film

68. The error in this radiograph can be corrected by changing the:
   a. vertical angulation
   b. horizontal angulation
   c. film placement
   d. film size

69. Which of the following would *not* likely be a reason for a film to appear completely clear?
   a. The film was not exposed.
   b. There was a power failure.
   c. The x-ray machine was not turned on.
   d. The film packet was empty.

70. If a film appears light, it was:
   a. overexposed
   b. underexposed
   c. improperly placed
   d. the wrong size of film

71. If a film appears dark, it was:
   a. overexposed
   b. underexposed
   c. improperly placed
   d. the wrong size of film

72. What are the irregular radiopaque projections in the maxillary anterior region in the radiograph below?
   a. overhangs on composite restorations
   b. calculus
   c. periodontal pockets
   d. extended cementum

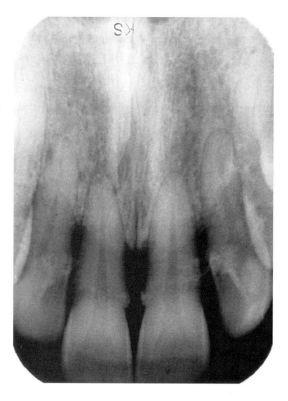

73. A healthy lamina dura in a radiograph will appear around the _____.
   a. apices of the tooth as a dense radiolucent line
   b. roots of the teeth as a radiolucent line
   c. apices of the tooth as a dense radiopaque line
   d. roots of the teeth as a dense radiopaque line

74. Digital radiography requires less radiation than conventional radiography because the:
   a. sensor is smaller
   b. sensor is more sensitive to x-rays
   c. exposure time is increased
   d. pixels sense transmitted light quickly

75. The image receptor found in the intraoral sensor is termed:
   a. CCD
   b. pixel
   c. semiconductor chip
   d. software

76. The method of obtaining a digital image similar to scanning a photograph to a computer screen is termed:
   a. direct digital imaging
   b. indirect digital imaging
   c. storage phosphor imaging
   d. pixel management

77. All of the following are advantages of digital radiography *except* _____.
   a. digital subtraction
   b. the ability to enhance the image
   c. size of the intraoral sensor
   d. patient education

78. A form of enhancement of the digital diagnostic image that is available for use is:
   a. transparency
   b. digital subtraction
   c. digital scanning
   d. storage phosphor imaging

79. _____ is an image receptor found in the intraoral sensor.
   a. Digitizer
   b. Pixel
   c. Sensor coupler
   d. Charge-coupled device

80. A _____ is a small detector that is placed intraorally to capture the radiographic image.
   a. charge-coupled device
   b. sensor
   c. pixel
   d. film block

81. To _____ is to convert an image into digital form that in turn can be processed by a computer.
- **a.** store
- **b.** detect
- **c.** digitize
- **d.** reflect

82. A tooth that has been torn away or dislodged by force.
- **a.** intrusion
- **b.** extrusion
- **c.** avulsion
- **d.** fracture

83. _____ resorption is a process seen with the normal shedding of primary teeth.
- **a.** External
- **b.** Internal
- **c.** Pathologic
- **d.** Physiologic

84. _____ is a diffuse calcification of the pulp chamber and pulp canals of teeth.
- **a.** Internal resorption
- **b.** Pulpal obliteration
- **c.** Pulpal sclerosis
- **d.** Pulp stones

85. Pulp stones _____ cause symptoms and _____ require treatment.
- **a.** do, do
- **b.** do, do not
- **c.** do not, do
- **d.** do not, do not

86. Which of the following is a periapical radiolucency?
- **a.** condensing osteitis
- **b.** hypercementosis
- **c.** periapical cyst
- **d.** sclerotic cyst

87. The periapical granuloma:
- **a.** refers to a tooth with an infection in the pulp
- **b.** is a purulent inflammation within the periodontal tissues
- **c.** is treated with deep scaling and debridement
- **d.** both b and c

88. Condensing osteitis is seen _____ the apex of a _____ tooth.
- **a.** below, vital
- **b.** below, nonvital
- **c.** above, vital
- **d.** above, nonvital

89. Which of the following statements is *not* true of the properties of x-rays?
    a. X-rays are invisible.
    b. X-rays can penetrate opaque tissues and structures.
    c. X-rays travel in circuitous lines.
    d. X-rays can adversely affect human tissue.

90. _____ is a measurement of force that refers to the potential difference between two electrical charges.
    a. Exposure time
    b. Wavelength
    c. Voltage
    d. Milliamperage

91. Which of the following statements is *true* of the use of voltage in dental x-ray equipment?
    a. Dental x-ray equipment requires the use of 3 to 5 V.
    b. Dental x-ray equipment requires the use of less than 65 kV.
    c. Dental x-ray equipment requires the use of more than 100 kV.
    d. Dental x-ray equipment requires the use of 65 to 100 kV.

92. When contrasted with the use of 65 to 75 kV for dental x-rays, the use of 85 to 100 kV produces:
    a. more penetrating dental x-rays with longer wavelength
    b. less penetrating dental x-rays with longer wavelength
    c. more penetrating dental x-rays with shorter wavelength
    d. less penetrating dental x-rays with shorter wavelength

93. _____ is the overall darkness or blackness of a radiograph.
    a. Contrast
    b. Density
    c. Gray scale
    d. Exposure

94. If the radiograph is not exposed for a sufficient amount of time or with a low _____ setting, the resulting radiograph will not have the correct overall _____ or will be light in appearance.
    a. mA, contrast
    b. kVp, density
    c. mA, density
    d. kVp, contrast

95. Which of these is *not* a factor that influences the density of a radiograph?
    a. distance from the x-ray tube to the patient
    b. developing time and temperature
    c. body size of the patient
    d. age of the patient

96. Which of the following organs is *not* considered a critical organ that is more sensitive to radiation?
    a. skin
    b. stomach
    c. thyroid gland
    d. lens of the eye

97. The purpose of the aluminum filter in the x-ray tubehead is to remove the _____energy, _____ wavelength, least penetrating x-rays from the beam.
 a. high, short
 b. low, long
 c. high, long
 d. low, short

98. Cortical bone is also referred to as '_____ bone.
 a. compact
 b. cancellous
 c. spongy
 d. trabecular

99. What is the landmark indicated by the arrows in the radiograph below?
 a. coronoid process ✓
 b. condyle
 c. internal oblique ridge
 d. zygomatic process of the maxilla ✓

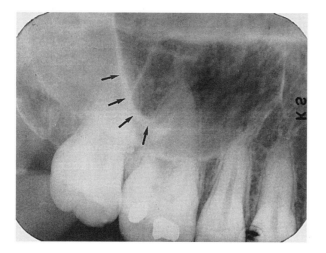

100. Which is *not* information found on a film mount?
 a. name of radiographer
 b. date of processing
 c. patient's full name
 d. dentist's name

Infection Control

Directions: Select the response that best answers each of the following questions. Only one response is correct.

1. If you opt not to receive a hepatitis B vaccination and have signed a waiver to this effect, you have the right to:
   a. change your mind and have the vaccination at your own expense ·
   b. change your mind and the employer is required to provide the vaccination
   c. demand periodic blood tests to ensure noninvasion of the hepatitis B virus in your body
   d. sue the employer if you contact hepatitis B

2. All dental professionals must use surgical masks and protective eyewear to protect the eyes and face:
   a. only during surgical procedures
   b. whenever the high-speed handpiece is used
   c. whenever spatter and aerosolized sprays of blood and saliva are likely
   d. if desired

3. All dental assistants involved in the direct provision of patient care must undergo routine training in:
   a. infection control, safety issues, and hazard communication
   b. charting, taking patients vital signs, and using the office intercom system
   c. infection control, uniform sizing, and ordering of disposables
   d. hazardous waste management, charting, and application of dental dam

4. When immunity is present at birth, it is referred to as:
   a. acquired immunity
   b. active immunity
   c. artificially acquired immunity
   d. inherited immunity

5. _____ immunity occurs when a vaccination is administered and the body forms antibodies in response to the vaccine.
   a. Active natural
   b. Active artificial
   c. Passive natural
   d. Passive artificial

6. A chronic infection is best exemplified by which of the following?
   a. hepatitis C virus
   b. cold sore
   c. common cold
   d. pneumonia

7. Which of the following exemplifies an acute infection?
   a. hepatitis C virus
   b. hepatitis B virus
   c. common cold
   d. pneumonia

8. Microorganisms that produce disease in humans are known as:
   a. nonpathogenic
   b. pathogens
   c. pasteurized
   d. germs

9. Bacteria can be identified by shape. Which of the following is a shape of bacteria?
   a. spherical (cocci)
   b. rod (bacilli)
   c. spiral (spirochetes)
   d. all of the above

10. An infection that results from a defective immune system that cannot defend against pathogens normally found in the environment is a(n):
   a. chronic infection
   b. latent infection
   c. acute infection
   d. opportunistic infection

11. A disease that can be transmitted in some way from one host to another is a(n):
   a. infectious disease
   b. communicable disease
   c. contagious disease
   d. all of the above

12. The transmission of a disease to a susceptible person by handling contaminated instruments or by touching contaminated surfaces is referred to as:
   a. airborne transmission
   b. direct transmission
   c. indirect transmission
   d. spatter transmission

13. Which of the following would be considered the best method for determining whether there is proper sterilization function of a sterilizer?
   a. a chemically treated tape used on packages that changes color
   b. the time, temperature, and pressure used
   c. a biological spore test through a monitoring system

14. When the assistant prepares a package of hazardous infectious waste for disposal, which of the following should be considered?
   a. All infectious waste destined for disposal should be placed in closable, leak-proof containers or bags that are color-coded or labeled appropriately.
   b. Infectious waste should be burned in a local incinerator.
   c. Only the clinical assistant should manage the removal of infectious waste.

15. Which of the following PPE is removed first after the completion of a clinical procedure?
   a. gloves
   b. protective eyewear
   c. gown
   d. mask

16. Exam gloves used during dental treatment can be made of:
   a. latex
   b. vinyl
   c. clear plastic
   d. a and b

17. Infectious or regulated waste (biohazard) include all of the flowing except:
   a. blood and blood-soaked materials ·
   b. pathologic waste ·
   c. sharps
   d. used barriers

18. Which of the following statements is *not* true as they apply to the use of overgloves?
   a. Overgloves must be worn carefully to avoid contamination during handling with contamination procedure gloves.
   b. Overgloves are placed before the secondary procedure is performed and are removed before patient treatment is resumed.
   c. Overgloves are discarded after a single use.
   d. Overgloves are acceptable alone as a hand barrier in nonsurgical procedures.

19. During which of the following procedures would you use sterile surgical gloves?
   a. placement of a composite
   b. periodontal surgery
   c. all bonding procedures
   d. removal of a suture

20. The most common route of disease transmission in the dental office is through:
   a. droplet infection
   b. direct contact with the patient's blood or saliva
   c. indirect contact with surfaces
   d. any instrument used intraorally

21. The strength of an organism in its ability to produce disease is:
   a. virulence
   b. bioburden
   c. pathogens
   d. infectious disease

22. The use of a preprocedural mouth rinse can lower the number of microorganisms that may escape a patient's mouth through all of the following routes *except* _____.
   a. aerosols
   b. spatter
   c. direct contact
   d. indirect contact

23. _____ infection is the mode of disease transmission that involves large-particle droplet spatter. _____ infection involves minute particles that can remain in the air for hours and can be inhaled.
   a. Airborne, indirect
   b. Airborne, droplet
   c. Droplet, aerosol
   d. Airborne, direct

24. Pathogens that are carried in the blood and body fluids of infected individuals and that can be transmitted to others are referred to as:
   a. bloodborne
   b. parenteral
   c. virulent
   d. acquired

25. Recommendations concerning gloves would fall under which of the following categories of infection control practices that directly relate to dental radiography procedures?
   a. protective attire and barrier techniques
   b. hand washing and care of hands
   c. sterilization or disinfection of instruments
   d. cleaning and disinfection of dental unit and environmental surfaces

26. Protective clothing:
   a. must prevent skin exposure when contact with blood or other bodily fluids is anticipated
   b. must prevent mucous membrane exposure when contact with blood or other bodily fluids is anticipated
   c. should be worn home and laundered daily
   d. both a and b

27. When using medical latex or vinyl gloves, _____.
   a. gloves may be rewashed between patients and reused until damaged
   b. nonsterile gloves are recommended for examinations and nonsurgical procedures
   c. hands should not be washed before gloving
   d. hands should not be washed between patients

28. _____ is defined as the absence of pathogens, or disease-causing microorganisms.
   a. Antiseptic
   b. Antibiotic
   c. Antiinfective
   d. Asepsis

29. Antiseptic is:
   a. the absence of pathogens or disease-causing microorganisms
   b. a substance that inhibits the growth of bacteria
   c. the use of a chemical or physical procedure to inhibit or destroy pathogens
   d. the act of sterilizing

30. While taking a patient's health history, it is noted that there is a history of tuberculosis and the patient is currently experiencing symptoms of this disease. Which of the following would *not* be appropriate action in the office?
   a. The patient should be referred promptly for medical evaluation of possible infectiousness.
   b. Tell the patient you will not be able to treat him or her anymore.
   c. Defer elective treatment until a physician confirms that the patient does not have infectious tuberculosis.
   d. If urgent dental care must be provided for the patient, and it is determined there is an infectious tuberculosis, obtain care that can be provided in a tuberculosis isolation center.

31. When can a liquid sterilant/high-level disinfectant achieve sterilization?
   a. sterilization will occur only when the solution is used at temperatures above 121° C
   b. sterilization will occur when the solution is used only for the longer exposure times
   c. sterilization will occur as soon as the minimal exposure time is reached
   d. sterilization will occur only when the solution is used under pressure

32. Which of the following may be used for surface disinfectant in the dental office?
   a. iodophors
   b. ethyl alcohol
   c. isopropyl alcohol
   d. ammonia

33. Before dental x-ray films are exposed, the treatment area must be prepared using:
   a. antiseptic
   b. aseptic techniques
   c. sterilization of critical instruments
   d. low-level disinfectant

34. Manufacturers of sterilizers (autoclaves) set them to reach a maximum steam temperature of ___ degrees Fahrenheit and pressure of ___ pounds per square inch (psi).
   a. 500, 40
   b. 350, 10 to 25
   c. 250, 15 to 30
   d. 400, 25

35. According to CDC guidelines when transporting a biopsy specimen it should be:
   a. placed in a flexible, leakproof container with a plain label and marked *hazardous.*
   b. placed in a sturdy, leakproof container labeled with a biohazard symbol.
   c. placed in an OSHA approved container and handled only by a federally licensed handler.
   d. placed in a sterile saline solution and then in a sturdy, leakproof container labeled with a biohazard symbol.

36. Instruments must be absolutely dry or they will rust or have an ash layer when using which type of sterilization process?
   a. chemical vapor
   b. cold sterile
   c. steam autoclave
   d. flash sterilization

37. Which of the following are considered to be semicritical instruments in radiography?
   a. the exposure button
   b. the x-ray control panel
   c. the lead apron
   d. x-ray film holding device

38. Which of the following statements is *true* concerning cleaning and disinfection of the dental unit and environmental surfaces?
   a. An intermediate-level disinfectant is recommended.
   b. A low-level disinfectant is recommended.
   c. EPA-registered chemical germicides labeled as both hospital disinfectants and tuberculocidals are classified as low-level disinfectants.
   d. both a and c

39. This method of sterilization requires good ventilation.
   a. steam under pressure
   b. cold chemical/immersion disinfection
   c. unsaturated chemical vapor
   d. flash sterilization

40. When using this method of sterilization, the exposure time varies as to whether the instruments are wrapped or unwrapped.
   a. steam under pressure
   b. cold chemical/immersion disinfection
   c. unsaturated chemical vapor
   d. flash sterilization

41. From the list below, select the best procedure for caring for an explorer.
   a. steam under pressure with emulsion
   b. steam under pressure without emulsion
   c. sharps container
   d. spray/wipe/spray with surface disinfectant

42. From the list below, select the best procedure for caring for a mouth mirror.
   a. steam under pressure with emulsion
   b. steam under pressure without emulsion
   c. cold chemical/immersion
   d. spray/wipe/spray with surface disinfectant

43. From the list below, select the best procedure for caring for a pair of crown and collar scissors.
   a. steam under pressure with emulsion
   b. steam under pressure without emulsion
   c. cold chemical/immersion
   d. spray/wipe/spray with surface disinfectant

44. From the list below, select the best procedure for caring for a handpiece.
   a. steam under pressure with emulsion
   b. steam under pressure without emulsion
   c. cold chemical/immersion

45. From the list below, select the best procedure for caring for a saliva ejector.
   a. steam under pressure with emulsion
   b. steam under pressure without emulsion
   c. cold chemical/immersion
   d. discard

46. From the list below, select the best procedure for caring for a contaminated needle.
   a. steam under pressure with emulsion
   b. steam under pressure without emulsion
   c. sharp's container
   d. discard in biohazard container

47. From the list below, select the best procedure for caring for a pair of protective glasses.
  a. steam under pressure with emulsion
  b. steam under pressure without emulsion
  c. cold chemical/immersion
  d. spray/wipe/spray with surface disinfectant

48. From the list below, select the best procedure for caring for medicament bottles.
  a. steam under pressure with emulsion
  b. steam under pressure without emulsion
  c. discard
  d. spray/wipe/spray or wipe/wipe with surface disinfectant

49. Which type of sterilization used in the dental office requires the highest temperature?
  a. steam autoclave
  b. chemical vapor
  c. dry heat sterilization
  d. chemical liquid sterilization

50. Immersion in a chemical liquid sterilant requires at least ___ hour(s) of contact time for sterilization to occur.
  a. 1
  b. 10
  c. 5
  d. 24

51. Which of the following is *not* a recommended method for sterilizing dental handpieces?
  a. chemical liquid sterilization
  b. steam sterilization
  c. chemical vapor sterilization

52. The ideal instrument processing area should be:
  a. large enough for several assistants to work at one time
  b. dedicated only to instrument processing
  c. part of the treatment rooms and dental laboratory
  d. outside the dental suite

53. There are areas of the instrument processing facility that govern the workflow pattern. The processing should flow in a single loop from:
  a. dirty, to sterile, to storage
  b. dirty, to clean, to sterile, to storage
  c. dirty, to preclean, to clean, to storage
  d. dirty, to preclean, to clean, to sterilize, to storage

54. The purpose of a holding solution is to:
  a. clean instruments
  b. disinfect instruments
  c. prevent the drying of blood and debris on instruments
  d. sterilize instruments

55. The least desirable method of precleaning dental instruments is:
    a. hand scrubbing
    b. ultrasonic cleaning
    c. instrument washing machines
    d. rinsing in a holding solution

56. The ultrasonic cleaner should be cleaned and disinfected:
    a. every other day
    b. once a week
    c. at least once a day
    d. once every 28 days

57. After instruments have completed the cleaning cycle of the ultrasonic cleaner, they should be:
    a. bagged
    b. rinsed with clear water
    c. placed in the sterilizer
    d. stored

58. The ultrasonic cleaner:
    a. cleans and removes debris
    b. cleans and disinfects
    c. cleans and sterilizes
    d. prewashes

59. Why is it important to keep an MSDS for the liquid sterilant (e.g., glutaraldehyde) on file?
    a. it completes the history of all materials used in the office
    b. it provides information on how to protect against exposure to a chemical and what to do if an exposure occurs
    c. it updates the records for future inspections
    d. it will prevent an exposure

60. The process that kills disease-causing microorganisms, but not necessarily all microbial life, is called:
    a. precleaning
    b. sterilization
    c. disinfection
    d. cleaning

61. Spores of *Bacillus atrophaeus* are used to monitor which of the following types of sterilizers?
    a. steam under pressure
    b. dry heat
    c. unsaturated chemical vapor

62. Patient care instruments are categorized into various classifications. Into which classification would instruments such as surgical forceps, scalpels, bone chisels, and scalers be placed?
    a. critical
    b. semicritical
    c. noncritical

63. For which of the following is there *not* a vaccine?
   a. influenza
   b. hepatitis B
   c. tetanus
   d. strep throat

64. Which of the following is *not* one of the most common methods of heat sterilization used in the dental office?
   a. hot water sterilization
   b. steam under pressure
   c. chemical vapor sterilization
   d. dry-heat sterilization

65. *Legionella* bacteria can cause what type of disease in a susceptible person?
   a. liver damage
   b. pneumonia
   c. intestinal damage.
   d. skin disease

66. Nosocomial infections are commonly acquired in:
   a. a dental office
   b. any type of business office
   c. a hospital or other medical facility
   d. restaurants

67. According to OSHA, the dental assistant may do which of the following prior to depositing a contaminated needle in a designated puncture-resistant container?
   a. recap it
   b. bend it
   c. break it
   d. none of the above are acceptable according to OSHA

68. OSHA requires a *minimum* of training of dental personnel in all of the following areas *except* _____.
   a. the Bloodborne Pathogens Standard
   b. the Hazard Communication Standard
   c. specialty safety standards
   d. general safety standards

69. The goal of a sound infection control program is to reduce cross-contamination from all of the following *except* _____.
   a. patient to patient
   b. patient to dental team members
   c. dental team members to other patients
   d. the community health program to the dental practice

70. Which of the following statements is *true* as it relates to the environmental infection control in a clinical area?
   a. Change barriers daily.
   b. Avoid the use of carpet and cloth-upholstered furnishings.
   c. Use isopropyl alcohol on fixed surfaces.
   d. Avoid barriers on light handles.

71. The Organization for Safety and Asepsis Procedures (OSAP) identifies the classification of clinical touch surfaces to include which of the following?
    a. instrument trays, handpiece holders, and countertops
    b. light handles, dental unit controls, and chair switches
    c. unit master switch, fixed cabinetry, and patient record
    d. telephone, assistant stool, and fixed cabinetry

72. Which of the following is *not* an acceptable method of preventing surface contamination?
    a. Use a surface barrier.
    b. Wipe the surface with alcohol.
    c. Preclean and disinfect the surface between patients.
    d. Clean and disinfect the surface with an EPA-registered disinfectant product.

73. What are standard precautions?
    a. the concept that considers all patients to have infections with a bloodborne pathogen
    b. the use of the same infection control procedures for all types of health care facilities
    c. the concept that considers that blood and all patient body fluids are potentially infectious
    d. the use of only infection control procedures formally approved by a government agency

74. The best time to clean and disinfect a dental prosthesis or impression that will be processed in the office laboratory is:
    a. after it has had time to dry
    b. after it is in the laboratory
    c. when it is convenient
    d. as soon as possible after removal from the patient's mouth

75. A victim who feels the effects of a chemical spill immediately, with symptoms of dizziness, headache, nausea, and vomiting, is experiencing:
    a. chronic chemical toxicity
    b. acute chemical toxicity
    c. chemical resistance
    d. mild exposure

76. _____ is considered regulated waste and requires special disposal.
    a. Human tissue
    b. Food
    c. Saliva-soaked gauze
    d. Used anesthetic carpule

77. Repeated exposure to chemicals at low levels for extended periods of time can result in liver disease or brain disorders that would be examples of:
    a. chronic chemical toxicity
    b. acute chemical toxicity
    c. terminal chemical toxicity

78. How often should the dental assistant or office safety supervisor check the contents of the emergency kit to determine that the contents are in place and within the expiration date?
    a. weekly
    b. monthly
    c. biannually
    d. annually

79. The floor in the entry to the dental office was wet. A patient slipped on the floor during entry to the office. There was no signage to include a potential slippery floor. Which of the following would be *true*?
    a. The office owner is responsible for providing signage for potential dangerous situations.
    b. The office owner is not held liable since the entry is not part of the clinical area.
    c. The office owner is not held liable since the patient should have been able to see the wet area since he or she was not legally blind.
    d. The office owner does not fall under such regulations because of the number of employees.

80. Wastes are classified as hazardous if they are:
    a. ignitable
    b. ingestible
    c. ultrasonic
    d. plastic

81. All waste containers that hold potentially infectious materials must:
    a. have a red bag
    b. be labeled with the biohazard symbol
    c. have special disposal
    d. be labeled as infectious waste

82. Scrap dental amalgam should be collected and stored in:
    a. a designated, dry, airtight container
    b. an airtight container under photographer fixer
    c. an airtight container under water
    d. both b and c

83. Which government agency enforces the disposal of regulated waste?
    a. OSHA
    b. EPA
    c. CDC
    d. FDA

84. The OSHA Hazard Communications Standard requires employers to do all *except* which of the following?
    a. Tell employees about the identity and hazards of chemicals in the workplace.
    b. Implement a hazard communication program.
    c. Maintain accurate and thorough MSDS records.
    d. Submit annual urinalysis results of all employees.

85. Which of the following is the dental staff required to have available and know the location of in the event of a heart attack or closed or blocked airway?
    a. crash cart
    b. oxygen
    c. IV stimulants
    d. patient's medications

86. Hazard communication training must include all of the following *except* _____.
    a. hazards of chemicals and proper handling of chemicals
    b. the availability and access of MSDS to all staff
    c. an explanation of the labeling of hazardous chemicals
    d. waivers of hepatitis C vaccinations

87. A dental health care worker transfers a small amount of a glass ionomer cement into a smaller container for use on a patient at chairside. A new label must be placed on that container if:

  a. more material is required during the course of treating that patient

  b. the chemical material is not used up at the conclusion of an 8-hour work shift

  c. the patient recently tested positive for HIV

  d. no MSDS can be found on file for that material

88. Hazard communication training must be provided:

  a. for all new employees at the beginning of employment

  b. anytime a new hazardous material is introduced into the office

  c. annually

  d. a and c

89. When recapping the needle, the dental assistant should use any of the following methods *except* _____.

  a. a one-handed scoop method

  b. a mechanical device specifically designed to hold the needle for recapping

  c. any safety feature that is fixed, provides a barrier between the assistant's hands and the needle following use, and allows the assistant's hands to remain behind the needle

  d. a two-handed scoop method for maximum control

90. Which of the following is *not* considered a "sharp"?

  a. metal matrix band

  b. metal matrix retainer

  c. orthodontic wire

  d. needle

91. Which of the following is *not* a main concern as a microorganism in a dental unit water line?

  a. *Pseudomonas*

  b. *Legionella*

  c. *Mycobacterium*

  d. *Lactobacillus*

92. The ADA, OSAP, and CDC recommend that the dental assistant:

  a. flush the dental unit waterlines for 30 seconds each morning and again at the end of the day

  b. flush the dental unit waterlines for 30 seconds each morning and between patients

  c. flush the dental unit waterlines 60 seconds each morning and 30 seconds after treating an HIV-infected patient

  d. flush the dental unit waterlines for 30 seconds each hour of the day

93. Shortly after donning the required PPE, the dental health care worker notices the following symptoms: watering eyes, nasal congestion, sneezing, coughing, wheezing, shortness of breath, and even dizziness. This person may be experiencing which type of reaction?

  a. immediate hypersensitivity (type I)

  b. delayed hypersensitivity (type IV)

  c. intermediate hypersensitivity (type III)

  d. irritant dermatitis (ID)

94. Which of the following are the recommended five parts of the Hazard Communication Standard?
    a. written program, inventory of hazardous chemicals, inventory of dental instruments, proper labeling of containers, employee training
    b. written program, inventory of hazardous chemicals, MSDS for every chemical, proper labeling of containers, employee training
    c. written records of staff health histories, inventory of hazardous chemicals, MSDS for every chemical, proper labeling of containers, employee training
    d. written program, inventory of hazardous chemicals, MSDS for every chemical, staff hair or urinalysis reports, employee training

95. Which of the following statements is *not* true?
    a. AIDS is a worldwide problem.
    b. HIV causes AIDS.
    c. HIV is transmitted through casual contact.
    d. HIV testing is recommended 6 months after the last possible exposure to HIV.

96. Switching to instruments with large, round diameters and contra-angled shanks may _____ the symptoms associated with carpal tunnel syndrome.
    a. help reduce
    b. exacerbate
    c. have little effect upon
    d. have no effect upon

97. Which of these factors should *not* be practiced during the use of nitrous oxide during conscious sedation?
    a. maintain conversation with the patient
    b. use dental dam, where applicable
    c. use a scavenger system
    d. secure the patient mask

98. Distillation of water is a _____ process that may remove volatile chemicals, endotoxins, and some microorganisms.
    a. sterilization
    b. reverse osmosis
    c. purification
    d. radiation

99. Which of the following statements is *not* true regarding the use of biohazard warning labels?
    a. The label is fluorescent orange or red-orange.
    b. The word *biohazard* on a label must be affixed to containers of regulated wastes.
    c. A label must be placed on a refrigerator if it contains blood and other potentially infectious material.
    d. White or green bags may be substituted for labels.

100. OSHA requires the use of standard precautions for _____.
    a. HIV-infected or AIDS patients
    b. potentially disease-infected patients
    c. patients not of record
    d. all patients

Answer Keys and Rationales

TEST 1

General Chairside

1. The position of the body standing erect with the feet together and the arms hanging at the sides with the palms facing forward is referred to as the:

   b. The anatomic position refers to the body when it is in a vertical position, with the face and the palms of the hands facing forward. A resting or postural position is not a term used in anatomic descriptions, and the supine position places a person on the back with the face up.

2. In the illustration shown, Dr. Curtis was assisted by Debbie May Ross to complete operative treatment for this patient. What required data are missing from the chart?

   d. The space for the file number was left blank. To be a legal document, a number or "NA" for "not applicable" should be inserted. The date of the appointment and the initials of the dentist, and dental assistant performing the treatment must also be included.

3. The examination technique in which the examiner uses his or her fingers and hands to feel for size, texture, and consistency of hard and soft tissue is called:

   b. Palpation is the examination technique in which the examiner uses the fingers and hands to feel for size, texture, and consistency of hard and soft tissue. Detection is the act or process of discovering tooth imperfections or decay, while probing is using a slender, flexible instrument to explore and measure the periodontal pocket. The extraoral exam is a visual inspection of the landmarks outside the oral cavity.

4. Which type of consent is given when a patient enters a dentist's office?

   b. Implied consent refers to the duties or actions that flow automatically for the relationship between the patient and the dental professional. The patient gives implied consent when he or she enters the dentist's office, at least for the dental exam. This is not informed consent, which demands more disclosure on the part of the provider about the care given a patient.

5. Consent is:

   b. Consent is voluntary and consent is given by a patient when he or she agrees to accept what is planned or done for him or her by another person.

6. A patient's chart that denotes abnormally small jaws would indicate:

   a. The word can be broken down into two parts: *micro,* meaning "small," and *gnathia,* meaning "jaw."

7. The tooth-numbering system that begins with the maxillary right third molar as tooth No. 1 and ends with the mandibular right third molar as tooth No. 32 is the:

   a. The Universal numbering system begins with the maxillary right third molar as tooth No. 1 and ends with the mandibular right third molar as tooth No. 32, whereas the other systems use either brackets or other numeric patterns to denote tooth numbering.

8. An abbreviation used in the progress notes or chart to indicate a mesioocclusobuccal restoration would be:

   d. Each surface is given an initial, and in the naming of this restoration, the surfaces are in the sequence of *mesial*, *occlusal*, and *buccal*—thus, MOB.

9. A hereditary abnormality in which there are defects in the enamel formation is:

   d. Amelogenesis refers to the formation of enamel, and imperfecta, an abnormality.

10. Any tooth that remains unerupted in the jaw beyond the time at which it should normally erupt is referred to as being:

   b. An impacted tooth is one that is so positioned in the jaw bone that eruption is not possible.

11. An oral habit consisting of involuntary gnashing, grinding, and clenching of the teeth is:

   b. Bruxism is the process of grinding the teeth; abrasion and attrition are both processes of wearing away of the tooth surface. Bulimia does not relate to these processes.

12. A horizontal or transverse plane divides the body into:

   a. When a body is divided horizontally, it will produce an upper and a lower portion or superior and inferior portions.

13. The cells associated with bone formation are known as:

   d. An osteoblast is a cell of mesodermal origin that is concerned with the formation of bone.

14. Which of the following teeth generally have two roots?

   b. All mandibular molars have two roots. Maxillary molars have three roots, whereas maxillary first premolars may have one or two roots.

15. Which of the following is *not* a function of the paranasal sinuses?

   c. There is no relationship with sinuses and digestion. Functions of the paranasal sinuses are to lighten the skull, provide resonance, and aid in warming respired air.

16. How many teeth are in the arch of a deciduous dentition?

   a. The deciduous dentition contains 20 teeth, 10 in each arch.

17. The tooth that has two roots and five cusps of which three are on the buccal and two are on the lingual would be a:

   c. The mandibular molars have two roots, and the maxillary first premolars may have one or two roots. The only mandibular molar with three buccal cusps on the buccal and two on the lingual is the first molar.

18. A 10-year-old patient would likely have which of the following teeth?

   a. At the age of 10 years, a child could have the permanent mandibular central and lateral incisors, primary second molars, permanent mandibular canines, and permanent first molars but would not yet have the permanent premolars or second molars.

19. What is the average range of the body's oral resting temperature?

   d. The normal adult body temperature is considered to be 98.6° F but may range between 97.6° F and 99° F.

20. The most common site for taking a patient's pulse in the dental office is the:

   c. The radial artery is the most common site for taking a patient's pulse in the dental office as it is readily accessible and accurate. The carotid or brachial would be an alternative if the pulse could not be obtained at the radial site.

21. The primary step in preventing a medical emergency is to be certain the patient has _____ before treatment is begun.

   c. It is necessary to obtain a complete medical history on each patient and at regular intervals to update this health history. Without an accurate and updated health history, the dental professional is unaware of potential health risks.

22. Which of the following is each member of the dental team *not* required to have the knowledge and skills to perform prior to handling an emergency in the dental office?
 b. Regulations do not require or permit all members of the dental health team to administer all cardiac medications.

23. The ABCDs of basic life support stand for:
 c. In all emergency situations, the rescuers must promptly initiate the ABCDs of basic life support: *airway, breathing, circulation, and defibrillation.*

24. The most frequently used substance in a medical emergency is:
 b. Glucose, epinephrine, and ammonia inhalants are included in an emergency kit, but oxygen is the most frequently used drug in a medical emergency.

25. The dental assistant's responsibility in an emergency situation is:
 d. The dental assistant works with the rest of the dental team to recognize the symptoms and signs of a significant medical complaint and to provide appropriate support in implementing emergency procedures. The dental assistant does not identify or diagnose a condition in the emergency situation.

26. _____, which is precipitated by stress and anxiety, may manifest in rapid, shallow breathing; lightheadedness; rapid heartbeat; and a panic-stricken appearance and is treated by having the patient breathe into a paper bag or cupped hands.
 b. When a patient is anxious or apprehensive, he or she may display rapid, shallow breathing; lightheadedness; rapid heartbeat; and a panic-stricken appearance. The patient is treated by breathing into a paper bag or cupped hands to increase the carbon dioxide supply and to restore the proper oxygen and carbon dioxide levels in the blood.

27. The list of emergency telephone numbers posted next to each telephone throughout the office should include all *except* _____.
 c. Patient emergency numbers are not posted in the office. Only those numbers that pertain to the office needs are posted near the telephone.

28. To ensure that a medical emergency is observed immediately, it is important for the dental assistant to:
 c. Because the dentist is concentrating on treatment in the oral cavity, the dental assistant needs to observe the patient throughout the procedure to note any changes in behavior or vital signs that would indicate potential medical complications.

29. The three characteristics noted in the patient record when measuring respirations are:
 b. The rate is the total number of breaths per minute, rhythm refers to the breathing pattern, and depth is the amount of air inhaled and exhaled during a breath.

30. The symbol on tooth No. 3 indicates that this tooth has a:
 a. The symbol "S" is a standard symbol indicating that a sealant has been placed on this tooth.

31. The symbols on teeth Nos. 18 through 20 indicate that:
 b. The symbols indicate that a bridge exists in this area and that tooth No. 19 is missing. Tooth No. 19 is a pontic, and teeth Nos. 18 and 20 are full gold crowns as abutments to the bridge.

32. Based on the chart given here, how many permanent teeth are present on the mandible?
 a. Permanent teeth Nos. 30, 26, 25, 24, 23, and 19 are all erupted.

33. When a patient's pulse is being taken, his or her arm should be:
 d. To ensure accurate measurement of the pulse, the arm should be well supported, extended and positioned at the same level or lower than the heart. To have the arm in a position that is not supported or above the heart will give an inaccurate reading.

34. Motion economy is the concept that encourages the dental health care worker to:
b. To conserve energy and increase productivity, motion economy is used to decrease the number and length of motions at chairside.

35. Which of the following devices might *not* be found on a prophylaxis tray?
c. All of the instruments except the fissure bur would be found on the prophylaxis tray. The fissure bur would be used in an operative procedure, not a prophylaxis.

36. Which of the following devices would be a choice for checking a patient's occlusion during an oral prophylaxis?
c. Articulating paper is a carbon-like paper that can make an imprint of the teeth during occlusal contact to identify the patient's bite pattern.

37. Which of the following should be done if the patient has thick, heavy saliva that adheres to the prophylaxis cup during the polishing procedure?
b. The HVE tip, when placed close to polishing cup, will prevent the thick, heavy saliva from adhering to the rubber cup, making it easier to polish the teeth. A saliva ejector is not strong enough to remove this heavy saliva.

38. What prosthetic device replaces missing teeth by metal framework and artificial teeth?
b. A mandibular partial denture is a type of restoration that has metal framework, acrylic, and artificial teeth. It replaces one or more teeth but not all of the teeth, as would a complete denture.

39. The portion of a bridge that replaces the missing tooth is called a(n):
c. The portion of the bridge that replaces the missing tooth is called the pontic, and the portion that is used for support or retention of the fixed prosthesis is the abutment.

40. Which of the following instruments would be used to measure the depth of the gingival sulcus?
a. The periodontal probe is designed with calibrations on the tip end to enable the operator to measure the depth of the gingival sulcus during routine examinations. The other instruments can identify dental anomalies but are not capable of measurement.

41. Which instrument is used to scale deep periodontal pockets or furcation areas?
b. The Gracey scaler is designed with multiple bends in the shank and a fine cutting edge to enable the tip to be placed into deep periodontal pockets and furcation areas.

42. The HVE system is used:
b. The HVE system is designed to remove large volumes of fluid and debris from the mouth during all operative and surgical procedures. The saliva ejector is a slow-speed evacuator and is not capable of removing debris from the mouth.

43. Which of the following instruments can be used to invert the rubber dam?
b. Although dental floss enables the operator to move the rubber dam into position at the interproximal surfaces of the tooth, the spoon excavator with the curved blade enables the operator to smoothly invert the rubber dam into the gingival sulcus. The explorer has a sharp pointed tip and could tear the dam and damage the soft tissue.

44. If treatment is to be performed on tooth No. 13, the following is true about clamp placement.
a. The general rule for rubber dam placement during an operative procedure is to place the clamp on the tooth distal to the last tooth being treated and then isolate the tooth being treated and the two teeth mesial to this tooth.

45. You are assisting a right-handed operator in a procedure performed on the patient's left side. The HVE tip and A/W syringe are being used. The operator signals for a transfer. You must:

b. In order for the assistant to pick up a new instrument to be transferred it will be necessary to transfer the A/W syringe to the right hand, retain the HVE tip in the right hand and pick up the new instrument to be transferred.

46. Which of the following is *not* a correct statement for seating the operating team?

c. The operator changes positions according to the arch being treated. The operator would never remain in the 12 o'clock position as it would interfere with the assistant and the mobile cart or tray.

47. When placing the amalgam into the preparation for a 31DO restoration, the first increment should be placed into the:

b. The first increment is placed into the proximal box as this is the most difficult area to gain access. Once the amalgam reaches the pulpal floor region, the amalgam can be packed into this area more easily.

48. Which of the following instruments would be used to grasp tissue or bone fragments during a surgical procedure?

a. The hemostat is a holding device that enables a person to grasp and clamp the tissue or material in place without fear of slippage. It is used often in surgery to grasp small tissue fragments to remove them from the region. A locking pliers does not have the grasping capability of the hemostat, and both of the other instruments are not used to grasp materials or tissues.

49. Which of the following is the common choice in providing for retention in a cavity preparation?

d. The small round bur, such as a No. ½, is a desirable bur to make a retentive groove. It forms a rounded surface on the cavity preparation floor to enable the material to lock in place.

50. Which of these would *not* be a form of matrix for an anterior esthetic restoration?

c. The universal metal matrix band is contraindicated for use with a composite type restoration, whereas the celluloid crown or strip is recommended.

51. When placing a composite restoration on the buccal cervical of tooth No. 30, which is the choice of matrix?

b. The Class V composite matrix is desirable because it is shaped in an oval form to replicate the shape of the cervical area of the tooth.

52. The most common form of anesthesia used in operative dentistry is:

a. Local anesthesia is used most often in operative dentistry. The other forms of anesthesia are used in specific situations but are not used commonly in operative dentistry.

53. For dental professionals, the safest allowable amount of N$_2$O is _____ parts per million.

a. For dental professionals, the safest allowable amount of N$_2$O is 50 parts per million. More than this amount in the dental environment may cause adverse effects.

54. Which of the following medical conditions is *not* a contraindication to using a vasoconstrictor in the local anesthesia during operative treatment?

d. Diabetes does not impact the administration of local anesthesia with a vasoconstrictor. The other conditions all relate to the circulatory system and may be impacted by the use of a vasoconstrictor in the local anesthesia.

55. _____ is frequently used on the mandibular teeth and is injected near a major nerve that anesthetizes the entire area served by that nerve branch.

a. Block anesthesia is the type of injection frequently required for most mandibular teeth and is injected near a major nerve. Block anesthesia numbs the entire area served by the nerve.

56. Nitrous oxide oxygen administration always begins and ends with:
   b. The patient is given 100% oxygen at the beginning of nitrous oxide administration to assist the dentist in determining the patient's tidal volume. Oxygenation at the end of the procedure helps to prevent a feeling of light headedness.

57. Which of the following is *not* a form of a retention aid for a crown when the tooth is extensively decayed, is fractured, or has had endodontic treatment?
   a. Resin-bonded brackets are not related to prosthodontic treatment, whereas the other responses are all forms of retention that may be used in the buildup of a tooth that has been extensively destroyed by disease or trauma.

58. The tray setup in the photograph is used to:
   d. The key instruments on this tray are the ligature ties, director, hemostat, and ligature cutter that are all related to the placement and removal of ligature ties. There are no bands or separators available.

59. To control swelling after a surgical procedure, the patient should be instructed to:
   a. Edema or swelling can best be reduced or kept to a minimum if the patient is directed to place a cold pack in a cycle of 20 minutes on and 20 minutes off for the first 24 hours. Heat is contraindicated for the reduction of swelling.

60. A painful condition that can occur after a surgical extraction is inflammation known as _____, also known as _____.
   b. Alveolitis, or dry socket, may occur after a surgical procedure due to the loss of the blood clot in the socket. This is a painful condition due to the exposure of nerve tissue.

61. It may take _____ to complete a dental implant procedure.
   c. Dependent on the complexity of the procedure and healing, it will take between 3 and 9 months to complete a dental implant procedure.

62. A metal frame that is placed under the periosteum and on top of the bone is called a(n):
   b. The prefix *sub* means "under" or "beneath" and thus identifies this answer as the subperiosteal implant since the metal frame is placed under the periosteum.

63. The natural rubber material used to obturate the pulp canal after treatment is completed is called:
   b. Gutta-percha is a natural rubber material used to obturate the pulpal canal after treatment has been completed. Neither hydrogen peroxide nor glass ionomer is used to obturate the canal.

64. In this photograph, which instrument is a barbed broach?
   a. The photograph in A illustrates the barbs that appear on a barbed broach.

65. A common solution used for irrigation during the debridement procedure in endodontic treatment is:
   c. Sodium hypochlorite, commonly referred to as bleach, is the common solution used for irrigating a canal during debridement. Sterile water and salt solutions are not used.

66. The incisional periodontal surgical procedure that does not remove tissues but pushes away the underlying tooth roots and alveolar bone is known as:
   c. In incisional surgery, also known as periodontal flap surgery or simply flap surgery, the tissues are not removed but are pushed away form the underlying tooth roots and alveolar bone.

67. Which of the following does *not* contribute to periodontal disease?
   d. Pathologic migration, bruxism, and mobility are all factors relating to periodontal disease, whereas the time a tooth erupts does not play a role in periodontal disease.

68. The _____ is an instrument that resembles a large spoon and is used to debride the interior of the socket to remove diseased tissue and abscesses.

   c. The surgical curette has two spoon-like tips that aid in debriding or cleaning out the interior surface of the socket following the removal of a tooth.

69. From the instruments shown here, select the curette.

   d. The photograph in D has two ends with spoon-like tips that are characteristic of a surgical curette.

70. Coronal polishing is a technique used for all of the following purposes *except* _____.

   c. The functions of coronal polishing are to remove plaque and stains from coronal surfaces of the teeth, before placement of dental sealants and orthodontic bands, and before placing dental dam and acid etching. Coronal polishing is not capable of removing calculus from subgingival surfaces.

71. Exogenous stains are caused by an environmental source and are classified into subdivisions, including which of the following?

   e. Dental stains are categorized as either endogenous or exogenous in nature. Exogenous stains are subdivided into extrinsic and intrinsic stains.

72. For which purpose is disclosing solution *not* used?

   b. Disclosing solution does not have the capability of desensitizing tissues. It is used only to identify the presence of plaque, show intrinsic stains, and evaluate the effectiveness of polishing or brushing.

73. The first step in placing dental sealants is to _____ the surface.

   c. Before a sealant can be placed, the tooth surface must be adequately cleaned.

74. Enamel that has been etched has the appearance of being:

   a. When the enamel has been etched appropriately, it will have a chalky appearance and will not be shiny, wet, or slightly discolored.

75. According to Black's classification of cavities, the type of decay diagnosed on the incisal edge of anterior teeth and the cusp tips of posterior teeth is _____.

   a. Class VI decay is caused by abrasion and defects, and it is diagnosed on the incisal edge of anterior teeth and the cusp tips of posterior teeth.

76. The isolation of multiple anterior teeth with a dental dam is usually placed _____.

   c. To adequately isolate the anterior region when more than one tooth is being treated, it is recommended that teeth from first premolar to first premolar be isolated. By isolating from first premolar to first premolar stability to the rubber dam will exist during isolation.

77. When one or more teeth are missing from the same quadrant, a permanent _____ would most commonly be recommended by the dentist.

   d. A fixed bridge can be placed when one or more teeth are missing from the same quadrant. This device cannot be removed by the patient.

78. Gingival retraction cord is placed _____ the crown preparation is completed and is removed _____ the final impression is taken.

   d. Prior to taking the final impression after the crown preparation is completed, retraction cord is placed into the gingival sulcus to enable retraction of the soft tissue. The impression will more adequately include the cervical margin of the preparation.

79. A _____ is an orthodontic _____ that is a custom appliance made of rubber or pliable acrylic that fits over the patient's dentition after orthodontic treatment.

   d. The Hawley appliance is the most commonly used removable custom-made appliance that is used as a positioner. It is worn to passively retain the teeth in their new position after the removal of the fixed appliances.

80. This tray setup is for:
   b. The setup includes elastometric ties, hemostat, and orthodontic scaler, all instruments used in placing and removing elastometric ties. There are no bands, arch wires, or separators present.

81. Instrument "A" in the photograph is used to:
   b. The instrument is a band seater and, when the patient bites gently onto it, aids the operator in forcing the band down onto approximately the middle third of the tooth.

82. A(n) _____ is used to provide interproximal space for inserting an orthodontic band.
   c. When a tight interproximal contact exists, it makes it impossible to properly seat an orthodontic band. Therefore, a separator is used for this purpose, to open up the contacts for inserting an orthodontic band.

83. _____, also known as *tongue tied,* results in a short lingual frenum.
   c. Ankyloglossia results in a short lingual frenum.

84. _____ is a condition in which an inflammation is uncontrolled within a localized area and spreads throughout the soft tissue and organ.
   b. Cellulitis is an uncontrollable inflammation that can spread throughout the soft tissue and organ.

85. _____ is a superficial infection caused by a yeast-like fungus.
   c. Oral candidiasis, a common opportunistic infection found in the oral cavity, is caused by yeast. Yeast is a form of fungi.

86. Which instrument would be used to remove the right mandibular first molar?
   a. The larger beaks will enable the operator to grasp the molar more readily than the other forceps, which is used for an anterior tooth.

87. Which instrument would be used to remove the right maxillary second molar?
   a. The forceps in B and C are both used for the mandible because their beaks are at nearly right angles to the handles. The forceps in A are for the maxillary molar. Their beaks are more nearly parallel to the handles and enable the operator to use them on the maxilla.

88. Using Black's classification of cavities, a lesion on the cervical third of a tooth is considered a Class _____ restoration or cavity.
   d. Carious lesions found on the cervical third of the tooth are classified as Class V in Black's classification.

89. Which of the following teeth are not succedaneous?
   c. A succedaneous tooth is one that replaces a primary tooth. There is no primary tooth found in the position of the permanent first molar. This tooth erupts behind the most distal primary molar.

90. The automatic external defibrillator (AED) is used for all *except* _____.
   b. The AED is basically an advanced computer microprocessor that assesses the patient's cardiac rhythm and identifies any rhythm for which a shock is indicated. The shock is a massive jolt of electricity that is sent to the heart muscle to reestablish the proper rhythm of the heart.

91. Which of the following is *not* a characteristic that allows dental materials to withstand the oral environment?
   d. Trituration and amalgamation are not characteristics of a dental material but rather a process of manipulating amalgam.

92. A dental restorative material that is applied to a tooth or teeth while the material is pliable and can be adapted, carved, and finished is classified as:
   a. A direct restoration is one that is placed and carved in the tooth during a single appointment. An indirect restoration requires an impression of the prepared tooth, and then a restoration such as a crown, bridge, or onlay is made outside the mouth and cemented into the tooth at another appointment or later time.

93. Which of these would have the least dimensional stability?
   c. Alginate hydrocolloid is subject to syneresis and imbibition due to the water content of the product. Thus, the dimensional stability of the material is very low.

94. The conventional or traditional composites, which contain the largest filler particles and provide the greatest strength, are known as:
   d. Macrofilled composites contain the largest of the filler particles, providing the greatest strength but resulting in a duller, rougher surface. Macrofilled composites are used in areas where greater strength is required to resist fracture.

95. If a light bodied impression catalyst is mixed with a heavy bodied impression base, the resultant mix might:
   b. The bases and catalysts of each consistency are chemically manufactured to work with the matched base or catalyst. If the base and catalyst is interchanged with the consistency tubes, the end result will not be accurate.

96. Addition of cold water to an alginate mix will cause the setting time to be:
   a. When cooler temperature water is used, it will take the mix longer to set; thus, the setting time is increased.

97. Select two terms that describe the purpose and consistency of a dental cement used for the final seating of a porcelain fused-to-metal crown.
   d. The final seating of a porcelain fused to metal crown requires a cement base that is of luting or primary consistency, which strings for about 1 inch. The purpose of seating the crown is for final cementation.

98. Noble metals used in indirect restorations include all *except* _____.
   c. Noble metals used for cast restorations are gold, palladium, and platinum.

99. Which of the following statements is *not* true about the use of calcium hydroxide as a frequently selected cavity liner?
   c. The other statements all identify the function of calcium hydroxide as a dental liner. Cost is not a characteristic considered in using calcium hydroxide as a liner.

100. The advantage of using a glass ionomer restorative material is:
   b. Fluoride release is a primary characteristic of glass ionomers and thus makes it a desirable restorative material.

101. A custom tray is constructed to fit the mouth of a specific patient and is used to _____, _____, and _____.
   b. When a custom tray is designed for a patient, it will adapt to the patient's mouth, fit around any anomalies, and reduce the amount of impression material needed.

102. Which form of gypsum product is commonly used for making diagnostic models?
   a. Plaster is the most porous of the gypsum products and is cost effective for use in the construction of diagnostic models.

103. When taking impressions, the next step after seating the patient and placing the patient napkin is to:
   c. Prior to taking impressions, the patient must be informed of the procedure and the process explained so that there is complete cooperation.

104. Prior to handing a record to the administrative assistant after treating a patient, the clinical assistant should:
   c. The clinical assistant must remove the gloves used during the clinical procedure and wash the hands prior to transporting the chart to the business assistant. This will avoid cross-contamination.

105. The information in a registration form should include all *except* _____.
   d. It is not pertinent information to include the age of all dependents. Vital information about the patient will include name, address, contact telephone numbers, place of employment of the responsible party, and information concerning the patient's insurance coverage.

106. Financial arrangements for treatment should *not* be made:
   c. Good business practice mandates that financial arrangements must be made prior to beginning the treatment for the patient.

107. _____ pay is the amount the dental assistant takes home after all the deductions are made.
   b. Net pay is the amount the earner receives in the payroll check. This amount equals the amount of the gross pay minus all deductions.

108. _____ is another name for the Social Security funds deducted from an employee's pay.
   b. Federal Insurance Contributions Act (FICA), commonly known as Social Security, is the amount the employer is required to deduct from the employee's gross income.

109. Which of these is an expendable item used in the dental office?
   c. An expendable item is a single-use item and is discarded after the single use.

110. Which is a capital item in a dental office?
   c. A capital item is one of great cost, generally over $1000, and will be reused for several years.

111. Oxygen should be stored:
   b. Oxygen tanks are always stored upright and secured tightly in place.

112. An office system that tracks patients' follow-up visits for an oral prophylaxis is a(n):
   c. A recall system is used to recall patients to the office for routine oral prophylaxis and may also be used in specialty offices for other recall treatment.

113. Which of the following statements should be reworded on a patient's record to avoid litigation?
   c. This statement is insensitive to the patient's reactions and could be an issue in any potential litigation.

114. What are the consequences of using a nickname or an incorrect name when filing an insurance claim form?
   b. If an insurance company does not have the accurate name of a patient, it will take longer to process a claim.

115. An administrative assistant records information the dentist dictates for a patient's clinical record after the treatment is complete. Later, litigation is taken against the dentist in the practice for treatment that was rendered. The administrative assistant is asked to testify. Which of the following statements is *true*?
   c. The administrative assistant is not an expert witness in clinical treatment and in this case can only testify that he or she did write the information that was dictated.

116. When speaking to a patient on the telephone, which is the most courteous action?
   b. Always wait for the patient to hang up. It may be possible that the patient has another question that needs to be answered.

117. The leading cause of tooth loss in adults is:
   c. Periodontal disease is the leading cause of tooth loss in adults. Almost 75% of American adults have some form of periodontal disease.

118. The first step in patient education is to:
   c. Before a dental health care professional can proceed in patient education, he or she must listen carefully to the patient; his or her needs and their understanding of their dental health care. This seems cumbersome now. Prior to beginning patient education, the dental health care professional should listen carefully to the patient to determine his or her needs and to determine their understanding of their dental health care.

119. The MyPyramid, formerly known as the Food Guide Pyramid, is an outline of what to eat each day. The largest section on the pyramid is in what food group?
  c. The base of the MyPyramid is composed of the bread, cereal, rice, and pasta group.

120. Which of the following statements is *false* regarding carbohydrates?
  d. Simple sugars are formed in the mouth from refined carbohydrates such as sugar, syrup, jellies, and such. Complex carbohydrates are found in grains, vegetables, and fruits and are less cariogenic because they clear the mouth before they are converted into simple sugars that can be used by bacteria.

Radiation Health and Safety

1. Radiographs are used in an oral diagnosis to detect all of the following *except* _____.
  c. During oral diagnosis, malocclusion is identified visually when the patient bites together so that both the mandibular and maxillary teeth are in alignment or with the use of diagnostic models. This is not a function of a dental radiograph.

2. In the radiograph below, what is the lesion at the apex of the mandibular central incisor?
  a. The lesion on the central incisor is a well-defined round radiolucency that is a periapical cyst.

3. Commercially available barrier envelopes:
  b. Barrier envelopes that fit over intraoral films can be used to protect the film packets from saliva and minimize contamination after exposure of the film.

4. Preparation of supplies and equipment involves sterilizing which of the following items?
  b. The film-holding device can be sterilized, whereas the lead apron and PID must be disinfected. Film is not sterilized.

5. Exposed films should _____ dried and then placed in a _____ for transport to the darkroom for processing.
  d. Exposed films should be dried and then placed in a disposable container for transport to the darkroom for processing. This will aid in reducing disease transmission and ensure that the films stay dry.

6. When handling film with barrier envelopes, the barrier envelopes are opened with _____ hands and the films unwrapped with _____ hands.
  b. When handling film with barrier envelopes, the barrier envelopes are opened with gloved hands and the films unwrapped with nongloved hands because the outside of the barrier is contaminated.

7. Root fractures occur most often in the _____ region.
  a. Due to the positioning of the maxillary central incisors, they are more likely than the other teeth to be the first to fracture.

8. The _____ radiograph is the film of choice for the evaluation of mandibular fractures.
  d. The panoramic view is the choice for the evaluation of mandibular fractures as it allows the dental professional to view a large area of the maxilla and mandible on a single film. Thus, the detection of diseases, lesions, and conditions of the jaws can be readily identified.

9. Overlapped interproximal contacts result from:
  b. Overlapped contacts are caused by incorrect horizontal angulation. The central ray has not been directed through the interproximal spaces; thus, the proximal surfaces of adjacent teeth appear overlapped and prevent the examination of the interproximal areas.

10. The quality of the x-ray photos is determined by the:
   a. In dental radiography, the term *quality* is used to describe the mean energy or penetrating ability of the x-ray beam. The quality or wavelength and energy of the x-ray beam is controlled by the kilovoltage.

11. When using the bisecting method the object–film distance is kept to a _____.
   b. The object-film distance is the distance between the object being radiographed (the tooth) and the dental x-ray film. The tooth and the x-ray film should always be placed as close together as possible. The closer the film to the tooth, the less image enlargement there will be on the film.

12. The advantage of double-emulsion intraoral films over the old single emulsion films is:
   c. Double-emulsion film is used instead of single-emulsion film (emulsion on one side only) because it requires less radiation exposure to produce an image.

13. Taking the film to be duplicated out of the mounts:
   c. By removing the films from the x-ray mount, it is possible to make better contact between the x-rays and the duplicating film. Without good contact, the duplicate film will appear fuzzy and show less detail than the original film.

14. A tissue that lies within the primary dental beam and receives a lot of secondary radiation is the _____.
   c. Critical organs exposed during dental radiographic procedures in the head and neck region include skin, thyroid gland, lens of the eye, and bone marrow.

15. Reticulation of the emulsion is usually the result of:
   d. A film will appear cracked when the temperature of the processing solution and water baths vary drastically.

16. All of the following affect the life of processing solutions *except* _____.
   d. The use of the safelight does not relate to the processing solutions.

17. If the manual developing time is 5 minutes, then the fixing time should be _____.
   d. Developing time of 5 minutes would indicate he solution temperature is 68° F and thus the time in the fixer would be 10 minutes according to standard time and temperature processing charts.

18. The protective coating on the emulsion is softened by the _____ and hardened by the _____.
   c. The purpose of the developer is to reduce the exposed, energized silver halide crystals chemically into black metallic silver. The developer solution softens the film emulsion during this process. After development, rinsing takes place and then fixing. This chemical solution removes the unexposed, unenergized silver halide crystals from the film emulsion. The fixer hardens the film emulsion during this process.

19. Barrier pack films should be used for:
   a. Barriers are part of Standard Precautions and are used for all patients to prevent the transmission of disease.

20. Dark films can be caused by:
   c. An overexposed film will appear dark and is caused by excessive exposure time, kilovoltage, or milliamperage or a combination of these factors.

21. In a full mouth survey:
   c. A full mouth survey or complete series of radiographs includes all of the tooth bearing areas of the upper and lower jaws. These regions include the dentulous areas that exhibit teeth as well as edentulous areas, or areas where teeth no longer are present.

22. An overexposed film will appear similar to an _____ film.
   a. Both the overexposed film and overdeveloped film appear dark. This is caused by excessive exposure time, kilovoltage, or milliamperage, or a combination of both of these factors; or excessive developing time.

23. Reversing the film to the x-ray beam will cause a _____.
    b. If a film is reversed in the patient's mouth during exposure, a herringbone pattern will appear on the processed film.

24. When using the bisecting techniques, the imaginary angle that is bisected is formed between the long axis of the tooth and the:
    c. The imaginary angle that is bisected is formed between the long axis of the tooth and the long axis of the film. It is the bisected angle at which the dental radiographer must direct the central beam of the x-ray beam in a perpendicular line.

25. The technique or concept that provides for the orientation of structures seen in two radiographs exposed at different angles to determine the buccal-lingual relationship of an object is referred to as the _____.
    c. The buccal object rule is used when it is necessary to establish a buccal-lingual position of a structure such as a foreign object or impacted tooth.

26. In the bisecting technique the tooth-film distance is:
    b. The film in the bisecting technique must be positioned to cover the prescribed area and be placed against the lingual surface of the tooth.

27. All bitewings are taken using the:
    a. In the bitewing technique, the film is placed in the mouth parallel to the crowns of both the upper and lower teeth.

28. The marked prominence that appears on a maxillary molar periapical film as a triangular radiopacity superimposed over, or inferior to, the maxillary tuberosity region is:
    c. The coronoid process is not seen on a mandibular periapical radiograph but does appear on a maxillary molar periapical film. The coronoid process appears as a triangular radiopacity superimposed over, or inferior to, the maxillary tuberosity.

29. The main disadvantage of panoramic films is:
    b. The images seen on a panoramic radiograph are not as sharp as those on intraoral radiographs because of the intensifying screens.

30. Which of the following methods is best for taking a radiograph of an impacted third molar on the mandible?
    b. This film allows for the evaluation of impacted teeth, fractures, and lesions located in the body of the mandible.

31. Cassettes with intensifying screens are used in extraoral radiography to _____.
    a. An intensifying screen is a device that transfers x-ray energy into visible light; the visible light, in turn, exposes the screen film. These screens intensify the effect of x-rays on the film and thus less radiation is required to expose a screen film, and the patient is exposed to less radiation.

32. A conventional panoramic projection will show both the right and left joints in the:
    a. A panoramic film shows a wide view of the upper and lower jaws in the lateral plane. In panoramic radiography, the film and tubehead rotate around the patient, producing a series of individual images that, when combined on a single film, create an overall view of the maxilla and mandible.

33. One advantage of the storage phosphor technique is that the sensor is:
    c. In the storage phosphor technique, the reusable imaging plate that is coated with phosphors is used and is more flexible and fits into the mouth more readily than the sensor with a fiberoptic cable.

34. The definition seen on a digital image compared with film is:
    c. At this time, image quality continues to be a source of debate. The resolution of an image is defined as the number of line pairs per millimeter (lp/mm). Conventional dental x-ray film has a resolution of 12 to 20 lp/mm. A digital imaging system using a CCD has a resolution closer to 10 lp/mm.

35. Three types of direct sensors are _____, _____, and _____.
    c. The systems listed are the three systems used in dentistry today. Some of the others listed do not exist. The three systems used today are the charge-coupled device (CCD), complementary metal oxide semiconductor (CMOS), and charge injection device (CID).

36. The main disadvantage of a metal rubber dam holder in endodontics is:
    d. Because the holder is metal, there will be a radiopaque image superimposed over the site of where the frame is placed.

37. On intraoral radiographs, when the patient's right is on your left, this is called _____ mounting.
    a. Labial mounting is the preferred method of mounting. The raised or convex side of the identification dot faces the viewer and then the films are viewed as if the viewer is looking directly at the patient; the patient's left side is on the viewer's right side and the patient's right side is on the viewer's left side.

38. On a routine full mouth survey, it is not possible to see the_____ foramen.
    d. Due to the location of the mandibular foramen, it is not possible to observe it on a routine FMS of radiographs.

39. It is difficult radiographically to differentiate dentin from:
    c. Dentin and cementum are not as radiopaque as enamel or as radiolucent as the pulp or bone.

40. Most lesions appear _____ on processed radiographs.
    b. As dental caries or other lesions are identified, they will appear radiolucent rather than radiopaque. As demineralization and destruction of the hard tooth structures take place, the tooth density in the area of the lesion allows greater penetration of x-rays in the carious lesion so that the lesion appears radiolucent or dark/black.

41. Caries that radiographically involve the dentin are classified as _____.
    d. Once the carious lesion passes through the Dentinoenamel Junction and invades the dentin, it is considered to be in an advanced stage.

42. An example of caries that is almost never seen on a radiograph is _____.
    c. It is not possible to easily distinguish lingual caries on a dental radiograph. This type of lesion is normally observed during the oral examination.

43. Temporary acrylic crowns appear _____ on radiographs.
    a. Acrylic resin restorations are often used as an interim or temporary crown or filling. Of all the nonmetallic restorations, acrylic is the least dense and appears radiolucent or barely visible on a dental radiograph.

44. Gold crowns appear _____ on radiographs.
    b. Gold crowns and bridges appear as large radiopaque restorations with smooth contours and regular borders.

45. Cement bases under restorations appear _____ on a radiograph.
    b. A base material appears radiopaque, but compared to amalgam, it is less radiodense and shows distinct margins.

46. Bitewing projections cannot be used to detect:
    c. Root fractures are not distinguishable on a bitewing projection because the entire root is not shown.

47. High pulp horns on teeth are usually associated with _____.
    b. As one ages, the pulp horns become less prominent.

48. Fractures of the mandible will appear:
    c. On a dental radiograph such as a panoramic view, a mandibular fracture appears as a radiolucent line at the site where the bone has separated.

49. Implants will appear _____ on radiographs.
    b. Metallic splints, plates, fixation screws, and stabilizing arches all appear radiopaque; their characteristic shape and size may vary.

50. To obtain the best definition of a suspected residual root tip, a _____ projection should be used.
    b. A periapical film will be adequate to detect the definition of a suspected residual root tip and will provide good dimension to the film.

51. A malignant tumor of bone will appear _____ on radiographs.
    b. All cysts and tumors seen in bone are radiolucent areas.

52. An enlarged and bulbous, or club shaped, root is usually a sign of _____.
    c. Hypercementosis is a condition characterized by the buildup of cementum on the root of the tooth. The buildup of cementum makes the root appear enlarged and bulbous, or club-shaped, instead of its usual conical appearance.

53. Treating a patient without proper radiographs is a breach of the _____.
    d. There are rarely any dental procedures that should be done without current and diagnostic radiographs because their use is now the accepted *standard of care*.

54. Original radiographs should always be kept in the:
    a. The original radiographs for a patient always remain in the dental office. Any transfers to a third party are done by making copies of the originals.

55. The concept that the dental practitioner should expose the patient to the least amount of radiation exposure within the dental office without excessive cost refers to the _____.
    b. In an effort to minimize the amount of radiation, the dental profession is guided by the ALARA principle, which means "as low as reasonably achievable."

56. The film below illustrates:
    d. This is a definite crease in the film resulting in a radiolucent line.

57. When a clear (unexposed) area appears on the film:
    a. This clear area indicates the PID was not directed at the center of the film and resulted in cone cutting.

58. When overlapped contacts appear on the film:
    b. Overlapped areas that appear on the film indicated the central ray was not directed through the interproximal spaces. The horizontal angulation was incorrect.

59. What is the problem with the molar bitewing?
    a. Third molar regions are not visible on this film. This is caused by incorrect film placement for the molar bitewing.

60. By changing the _____, the clinical value of this film could be improved.
    c. This is incorrect film placement. To prevent this error, make certain that the anterior edge of the bitewing film is positioned at the midline of the mandibular second premolar. Always center the molar bitewing on the mandibular second molar, even when no erupted third molars are present.

61. _____ is the error in the film below.
    c. This is incorrect film placement. To prevent this error, make certain that the anterior edge of the bitewing film is positioned at the midline of the mandibular canine.

62. The error in the radiograph below is:
    b. The clear area on the film is cone cutting and it is caused by the PID not being directed at the center of the film.

63. The error in the radiograph below is:
    a. This is incorrect film placement. The film was not positioned in the patient's mouth to cover the apical regions of the teeth. Make certain that no more than $\frac{1}{8}$ inch of the film edge extends beyond the incisal-occlusal surfaces of the teeth when placing the film for his periapical view.

64. The error in the radiograph below is:
b. The overlapped image is the result of incorrect horizontal angulation. To avoid overlapped contacts on a periapical film, direct the x-ray beam through the interproximal regions.

65. The error in this radiograph is:
b. This image is elongated.

66. The error in this radiograph is caused by incorrect:
a. This image is elongated and is caused by incorrect vertical angulation. To avoid elongated images, use adequate vertical angulation with the bisecting technique or use the Rinn-type instrument to minimize such errors with the paralleling technique.

67. The error in this radiograph is:
a. This image is foreshortened.

68. The error in this radiograph is caused by:
a. This image is foreshortened and is caused by incorrect vertical angulation. To avoid foreshortened images, do not use excessive vertical angulation with the bisecting technique or use the Rinn-type instrument to minimize such errors with the paralleling technique.

69. Which of the following would *not* likely be a reason for a film to appear completely clear?
d. If there was no film in the packet, there would be no image on the film.

70. If a film appears light, it was:
b. If a film is underexposed, it will appear light. The reverse is true if the film is overexposed.

71. If a film appears dark, it was:
a. If a film is overexposed, it will appear light. The reverse is true if the film is underexposed.

72. What are the irregular radiopaque projections in the maxillary anterior region in the radiograph below?
b. Calculus appears radiopaque (white or light) on a dental radiograph. It most commonly appears as pointed or irregular radiopaque projections extending from the proximal root surfaces.

73. A healthy lamina dura in a radiograph will appear around the _____.
d. On a dental radiograph, the lamina dura appears as a dense radiopaque line that surrounds the root of a tooth.

74. Digital radiography requires less radiation than conventional radiography because the:
b. Less x-radiation is required in digital radiography because the typical sensor is more sensitive to x-rays than conventional film.

75. The image receptor found in the intraoral sensor is termed:
a. The charge-coupled device (CCD) is one of the most common image receptors used in dental digital radiography.

76. The method of obtaining a digital image similar to scanning a photograph to a computer screen is termed:
b. Indirect digital imaging is the method of obtaining a digital image in which an existing radiograph is scanned and converted into a digital form using a CCD camera.

77. All of the following are advantages of digital radiography *except* _____.
c. Some digital sensors are thicker and less flexible than intraoral film. Patients may complain of the bulky nature of the sensor and the sensor may be uncomfortable or may cause a gag reflex.

78. A form of enhancement of the digital diagnostic image that is available for use is:
   b. With digital subtraction, the gray scale is reversed so that radiolucent images (normally black) appear white and radiopaque images (normally white) appear black. This process also eliminates distracting background information.

79. _____ is an image receptor found in the intraoral sensor.
   d. The charge-coupled device (CCD) is one of the most common image receptors used in dental digital radiography.

80. _____ is a small detector that is placed intraorally to capture the radiographic image.
   b. In digital radiography, a small detector, called a sensor, is placed intraorally to capture a radiographic image.

81. To _____ is to convert an image into digital form that in turn can be processed by a computer.
   c. To digitize in dental digital radiography is to convert an image into a digital form that in turn can be processed by a computer.

82. A tooth that has been torn away or dislodged by force.
   c. Avulsion is to have the tooth torn away or dislodged from force; intrusion is to have the tooth pushed into the socket; extrusion is to have the tooth pushed out of the socket; a fracture is a break in the tooth.

83. _____ resorption is a process seen with the normal shedding of primary teeth.
   d. Physiologic resorption is shedding of primary teeth. The roots of primary teeth are resorbed as the permanent successors move in an occlusal direction.

84. _____ is a diffuse calcification of the pulp chamber and pulp canals of teeth.
   c. Pulpal sclerosis is a diffuse calcification of the pulp chamber and pulp canals of teeth that results in a pulp cavity of decreased size.

85. Pulp stones _____ cause symptoms and _____ require treatment.
   d. Pulp stones are calcifications that are found in the pulp chamber or pulp canals of teeth. The cause of pulp stones is unknown and do not cause symptoms and do not require treatment.

86. Which of the following is a periapical radiolucency?
   c. Only the periapical cyst would demonstrate a radiolucency at the apex of the tooth.

87. The periapical granuloma:
   a. The periapical granuloma results from pulpal death and necrosis and is the most common sequelae of pulpitis. A periapical granuloma may give rise to a periapical cyst or periapical abscess.

88. Condensing osteitis is seen _____ the apex of a _____ tooth.
   b. Condensing osteitis is a well-defined radiopacity that is seen below the apex of a nonvital tooth with a history of longstanding pulpitis.

89. Which of the following statements is *not* true of the properties of x-rays?
   c. X-rays travel in a straight line not a circuitous line.

90. _____ is a measurement of force that refers to the potential difference between two electrical charges.
   c. Voltage is the term used to describe the electric potential or force that drives an electric current through a circuit.

91. Which of the following statements is *true* of the use of voltage in dental x-ray equipment?
   d. The dental x-ray machine uses both types of transformers, step up and step down, in taking ordinary line or house voltage of 110 V and stepping it up to a range of 65,000 to 100,000 V (65-100 kVp) in the high-voltage circuit or stepping line voltage down to 3 to 5 V in the filament circuit; these being the two basic circuits in the dental x-ray machine.

92. When contrasted with the use of 65 to 75 kV for dental x-rays, the use of 85 to 100 kV produces:
    c. The use of 85 to 100 kV produces more penetrating dental x-rays with greater energy and shorter wavelengths, whereas the use of 65 to 75 kV produces less penetrating dental x-rays with less energy and longer wavelengths.

93. _____ is the overall darkness or blackness of a radiograph.
    d. Density is the overall darkness or blackness of a radiograph.

94. If the radiograph is not exposed for a sufficient amount of time or with a low _____ setting, the resulting radiograph will not have the correct overall ____ or will be light in appearance.
    c. The exposure time, as with milliamperage, affects the number of x-rays produced. Milliamperage controls the penetrating power of the x-ray beam by controlling the number of electrons produced in the x-ray tube and number of x-rays produced. Higher milliamperage settings produce a beam with more energy, thus increasing the intensity of the x-ray beam and having an impact on density of the film.

95. Which of these is *not* a factor that influences the density of a radiograph?
    d. Each of the answers a through c affects the density of a radiograph except for age, which does not relate to the result of the final radiograph.

96. Which of the following organs is *not* considered a critical organ that is more sensitive to radiation?
    b. The stomach is not considered a critical organ as it relates to x-ray exposure.

97. The purpose of the aluminum filter in the x-ray tubehead is to remove the ____ energy, ____ wavelength, least penetrating x-rays from the beam.
    b. The function of the filter is to remove the low energy, longer wavelength x-rays from the beam. These x-rays are not useful in producing a diagnostic quality radiograph and are harmful to the patient.

98. Cortical bone is also referred to as _____ bone.
    a. The cortical or compact bone is the outer layer of bone that appears radiopaque.

99. What is the landmark indicated by the arrows in the radiograph below?
    d. This bony prominence is the zygomatic process of the maxilla.

100. Which is *not* information found on a film mount?
    b. The date of processing is irrelevant data. Commonly, films are processed on the day of exposure but this may be modified. The important date is the date of exposure.

Infection Control

1. If you opt not to receive a hepatitis B vaccination and have signed a waiver to this effect, you have the right to:
   b. In accordance with the OSHA Bloodborne Pathogens Standard, the employee who initially declines the vaccination may at a later date, while still covered under the standard, decide to accept the offer. The employer must make the vaccine available at no charge at that time.

2. All dental professionals must use surgical masks and protective eyewear to protect the eyes and face:
   c. In accordance with OSHA recommendations, surgical masks and protective eyewear are to be worn whenever splashes, spray, spatter, or droplets of blood or saliva may be generated and eye, nose, or mouth contamination may occur.

3. All dental assistants involved in the direct provision of patient care must undergo routine training in:
   a. The OSHA standard requires that employers shall ensure that all employees with occupational exposure participate in a training program on the hazards associated with body fluids, safety issues, hazard communication, and the protective techniques needed to be taken to minimize the risk of occupational exposure.

4. When immunity is present at birth, it is referred to as:
   d. When immunity is present at birth, it is called inherited immunity. Immunity that is developed during a person's lifetime is called acquired immunity.

5. _____ immunity occurs when a vaccination is administered and the body forms antibodies in response to the vaccine.
   b. When a human body has not been exposed to a disease, it has not developed antibodies and is completely defenseless against the disease. Antibodies can be introduced into the body artificially by immunization or vaccination. The body then forms antibodies in response to the vaccine, and this is known as active artificial immunity.

6. A chronic infection is best exemplified by which of the following?
   a. A chronic infection is one of long duration.

7. Which of the following exemplifies an acute infection?
   c. An acute infection is of short duration but may be severe.

8. Microorganisms that produce disease in humans are known as:
   b. A pathogen is a microorganism or substance capable of producing a disease.

9. Bacteria can be identified by shape. Which of the following is a shape of bacteria?
   d. Bacteria can be found in three shapes: spherical, rod, or spiral.

10. An infection that results from a defective immune system that cannot defend against pathogens normally found in the environment is a(n):
    d. An opportunistic infection results from a defective immune system that cannot defend against pathogens normally found in the environment. This infection is seen in patients receiving large doses of steroids or other immunosuppressive drugs or in patients with acquired immunodeficiency syndrome.

11. A disease that can be transmitted in some way from one host to another is a(n):
    d. All terms above identify a disease that can be transmitted in some way from one host to another.

12. The transmission of a disease to a susceptible person by handling contaminated instruments or by touching contaminated surfaces is referred to as:
    c. The indirect transfer of organisms to a susceptible person can occur by handling contaminated instruments or touching contaminated surfaces and then touching the face, eyes, or mouth.

13. Which of the following would be considered the best method for determining whether there is proper sterilization function of a sterilizer?
    c. Biological monitoring, or spore testing is the only way to determine if sterilization has occurred and all bacteria and endospores have been killed. The CDC, ADA, and OSAP all recommend at least weekly biologic monitoring of sterilization equipment.

14. When the assistant prepares a package of hazardous infectious waste for disposal, which of the following should be considered?
    a. When waste leaves the office, the EPA regulations apply to the disposal. All waste containers that hold potentially infectious materials, whether regulated or nonregulated, must be placed in closable, leak-proof containers or bags that are color-coded or labeled appropriately with the biohazard symbol.

15. Which of the following PPE is removed first after the completion of a clinical procedure?
  c. The gown is removed first by reaching back and pulling it over the gloves and turning it inside out.

16. Exam gloves used during dental treatment can be made of:
  d. Gloves used during routine examination and treatment may be made of vinyl or latex.

17. Infectious or regulated waste (biohazard) include all of the flowing except:
  d. Barriers used during treatment typically are not considered infectious waste, unless for some reason they become blood soaked.

18. Which of the following statements is *not* true as they apply to the use of overgloves?
  d. At no time would overgloves be an acceptable hand barrier. They are used only as an alternative to changing gloves in situations where you may need to leave the chair to obtain a material or enter a cabinet drawer and want to prevent contaminating an area without changing gloves.

19. During which of the following procedures would you use sterile surgical gloves?
  b. During invasive procedures, such as surgery, it would be necessary to wear sterile surgical gloves.

20. The most common route of disease transmission in the dental office is through:
  b. For the dental health team, the most common route of disease transmission is direct contact with the patient's blood or saliva.

21. The strength of an organism in its ability to produce disease is:
  a. After microorganisms enter the body, three basic factors determine whether an infectious disease will develop: virulence (the pathogenic properties of the invading microorganism, dose (the number of microorganisms that invade the body), and resistance (the body's defense mechanism of the host).

22. The use of a preprocedural mouth rinse can lower the number of microorganisms that may escape a patient's mouth through all of the following routes *except* _____.
  d. The indirect transfer of organisms to a susceptible person can occur by handling contaminated instruments or touching contaminated surfaces and then touching the face, eyes, or mouth. The oral mouthwash will not reduce microorganisms from this method of transmission.

23. _____ infection is the mode of disease transmission that involves large-particle droplet spatter. _____ infection involves minute particles that can remain in the air for hours and can be inhaled.
  c. Large particle spatter is referred to as droplet infection, whereas the small particle size droplet can remain in the air for hours and is referred to as airborne infection.

24. Pathogens that are carried in the blood and body fluids of infected individuals and that can be transmitted to others are referred to as:
  a. Bloodborne pathogens are disease producing microorganisms that are carried in the blood and body fluids of infected individuals and that can be transmitted to others.

25. Recommendations concerning gloves would fall under which of the following categories of infection control practices that directly relate to dental radiography procedures?
  a. The wearing of gloves during patient treatment is a standard precaution and one of the pieces of personal protective equipment (PPE).

26. Protective clothing:
  d. The OSHA Standard requires that protective clothing such as laboratory coats and jackets must be worn to prevent skin mucous membrane exposure when contact with blood or other bodily fluids is anticipated.

27. When using medical latex or vinyl gloves, _____.
    b. Nonsterile gloves are recommended for examinations and nonsurgical procedures. Sterile gloves are worn during invasive surgical procedures.

28. _____ is defined as the absence of pathogens, or disease-causing microorganisms.
    d. The term *asepsis* refers to a "sterile state; a condition free from germs, infection and any form of life."

29. Antiseptic is:
    b. *Antisepsis* means "anti" (against) + "sepsis" (putrefaction). This is the prevention of sepsis by preventing or inhibiting the growth of causative microorganisms. Thus, antiseptic is the substance that inhibits the growth of bacteria.

30. While taking a patient's health history, it is noted that there is a history of tuberculosis and the patient is currently experiencing symptoms of this disease. Which of the following would *not* be appropriate action in the office?
    b. The patient should not be told you are unable to treat him. Rather, arrangements should be made to determine the state of the disease and then defer any elective treatment until the patient has been released by the physician. Emergency dental care can be provided in an isolation setting.

31. When can a liquid sterilant/high-level disinfectant achieve sterilization?
    b. Sterilization will occur with a high-level disinfectant when the solution is used only for longer exposure times consistent with manufacturer's directions.

32. Which of the following may be used for surface disinfectant in the dental office?
    a. From this list, the iodophors would be the best choice for a surface disinfectant. It is a well-known killing agent but does have some undesirable properties of corrosiveness, irritation of tissues, and allergenicity.

33. Before dental x-ray films are exposed, the treatment area must be prepared using:
    b. As with all treatment prior to the procedure the treatment area must be prepared using aseptic techniques.

34. Manufacturers of sterilizers (autoclaves) set them to reach a maximum steam temperature of ___ degrees Fahrenheit and pressure of ___ pounds per square inch (psi).
    c. Most manufacturers preset the sterilizers to reach a maximum steam temperature of 250 to 260 degrees Fahrenheit and a pressure of 15 to 30 pounds per square inch.

35. According to CDC guidelines when transporting a biopsy specimen it should be:
    b. According to CDC guidelines when transporting a biopsy specimen it should be placed in a sturdy, leakproof container labeled with a biohazard symbol.

36. Instruments must be absolutely dry or they will rust or have an ash layer when using which type of sterilization process?
    a. When using the chemical vapor processing method for sterilizing instruments, it is absolutely necessary to dry the instruments or they will rust or have an ash layer left on the surface.

37. Which of the following are considered to be semicritical instruments in radiography?
    d. The CDC categorizes patient care items according to critical, semicritical, or noncritical based on the potential risk of infection during use of the items. An x-ray holding device is a semicritical item that is heat resistant and, at a minimum, must be cleaned and treated with a high-level disinfectant.

38. Which of the following statements is *true* concerning cleaning and disinfection of the dental unit and environmental surfaces?
    a. These surfaces fall into the noncritical items and are cleaned and treated with low-level disinfectant if no blood is visible on the item or an intermediate level disinfectant if blood is visible. The dental unit is subjected to aerosols and would be subjected to blood and saliva spatter; thus, the intermediate level of disinfection is necessary.

39. This method of sterilization requires good ventilation.

   c. The unsaturated chemical vapor system of sterilization requires good ventilation in the sterilization area due to possible vapors being released into the environment.

40. When using this method of sterilization, the exposure time varies as to whether the instruments are wrapped or unwrapped.

   d. Time will vary in flash sterilization due to whether the instruments are wrapped or unwrapped. The manufacturer's directions should be followed with each piece of equipment.

41. From the list below, select the best procedure for caring for an explorer.

   a. The sharp points on an explorer require that these tips be protected with an emulsion prior to steam under pressure sterilization.

42. From the list below, select the best procedure for caring for a mouth mirror.

   b. Emulsion on a mirror will possibly leave a film on the mirror and, thus, it can be sterilized under steam under pressure without an emulsion. The other two methods are not acceptable methods of sterilizing the mirror.

43. From the list below, select the best procedure for caring for a pair of crown and collar scissors.

   a. The sharp edges on the beaks of the scissors require that these beaks be protected with an emulsion prior to steam under pressure sterilization.

44. From the list below, select the best procedure for caring for a handpiece.

   b. Emulsion on a handpiece may conflict with the manufacturer's recommendations and, thus, most handpieces can be sterilized by steam under pressure without an emulsion. In all cases, the manufacturer's directions should be consulted prior to sterilizing a handpiece for the first time.

45. From the list below, select the best procedure for caring for a saliva ejector.

   d. Saliva ejectors are manufactured for a one-time use only.

46. From the list below, select the best procedure for caring for a contaminated needle.

   c. All needles are placed in a sharps container.

47. From the list below, select the best procedure for caring for a pair of protective glasses.

   c. Protective eyewear that is nonprescription is placed in cold chemical immersion to disinfect/sterilize.

48. From the list below, select the best procedure for caring for medicament bottles.

   d. Medicament bottles are reused at chairside and must be disinfected. This is best accomplished by spray/wipe/spray or wipe/wipe. If using a spray, the first spray/wipe is to clean and then the surface is sprayed a second time to disinfect, and it remains to dry. If using wipes, then the first wipe is to clean and the second wipe is to disinfect.

49. Which type of sterilization used in the dental office requires the highest temperature?

   c. Dry heat sterilization requires the highest degree of heat and the longest time.

50. Immersion in a chemical liquid sterilant requires at least ____ hour(s) of contact time for sterilization to occur.

   b. Immersion in a chemical liquid sterilant requires at least 10 hours of contact time for sterilization to occur according to most manufacturers.

51. Which of the following is *not* a recommended method for sterilizing dental handpieces?

   a. Handpieces are never placed in a chemical liquid sterilant because the internal parts would be damaged.

52. The ideal instrument processing area should be:

   b. To avoid disease transmission, the instrument processing area/sterilization area should be dedicated only to instrument processing.

53. There are areas of the instrument processing facility that govern the workflow pattern. The processing should flow in a single loop from:

   b. In designing an instrument processing area, the facility should flow in a single loop from dirty, to clean, to sterile, to storage.

54. The purpose of a holding solution is to:

   c. The holding (presoaking) process facilitates the cleaning process by preventing debris from drying on the instruments.

55. The least desirable method of precleaning dental instruments is:

   a. Hand washing must be avoided as it can potentially cause glove punctures and result in injury to the assistant.

56. The ultrasonic cleaner should be cleaned and disinfected:

   c. Each day the ultrasonic cleaner is cleaned and disinfected before using it the next day to provide a clean tank for processing the next day's instruments.

57. After instruments have completed the cleaning cycle of the ultrasonic cleaner, they should be:

   b. Instruments are placed in the ultrasonic cleaner for the appropriate time and then rinsed thoroughly prior to the next steps in processing.

58. The ultrasonic cleaner:

   a. The ultrasonic cleaner does only cleaning; it does not disinfect or sterilize.

59. Why is it important to keep an MSDS for the liquid sterilant (e.g., glutaraldehyde) on file?

   b. The MSDS sheet provides valuable information on how to manage an exposure should one occur.

60. The process that kills disease-causing microorganisms, but not necessarily all microbial life, is called:

   c. Disinfection is capable of destroying some microorganisms but not all microbial life. Therefore, when possible, all items that can be should be sterilized or discarded.

61. Spores of *Bacillus atrophaeus* are used to monitor which of the following types of sterilizers?

   b. Biologic indicators contain the bacterial endospores used for monitoring. The spores used are *Geobacillus stearothermophilus* for steam under pressure and *Bacillus atrophaeus* for dry heat.

62. Patient care instruments are categorized into various classifications. Into which classification would instruments such as surgical forceps, scalpels, bone chisels, and scalers be placed?

   a. All of these instruments are in the critical category as they are used in invasive procedures and must be cleaned and sterilized by heat.

63. For which of the following is there *not* a vaccine?

   d. Strep throat is a disease for which a person is not vaccinated. For each of the other diseases, there is some form of vaccine.

64. Which of the following is *not* one of the most common methods of heat sterilization used in the dental office?

   a. Hot water is not an option for sterilization. Steam sterilization, using distilled water, must be under pressure to be effective.

65. *Legionella* bacteria can cause what type of disease in a susceptible person?

   b. This bacteria occurs naturally in water and may be resistant to some chlorines in domestic water as they can exist inside certain free-living amoebae as the causative agent of a type of pneumonia called Legionnaires' disease.

66. Nosocomial infections are commonly acquired in:

   c. Nosocomial infections are those infections commonly acquired in a hospital or medical setting.

67. According to OSHA, the dental assistant may do which of the following prior to depositing a contaminated needle in a designated puncture-resistant container?
   a. Needles are recapped in a recapping device at chairside after being used and then discarded in the sharps container.

68. OSHA requires a *minimum* of training of dental personnel in all of the following areas *except* _____.
   c. OSHA requires that an employee receive training in the Bloodborne Pathogens Standard, the Hazard Communication Standard, and general safety standards.

69. The goal of a sound infection control program is to reduce cross-contamination from all of the following *except* _____.
   d. A sound infection control program seeks to reduce cross-contamination in all of the above except a community health program to the dental practice that is not a viable recognized program.

70. Which of the following statements is *true* as it relates to the environmental infection control in a clinical area?
   b. Hard surfaces are much easier to maintain and do not collect debris and materials; thus, carpet and cloth-upholstered furnishings in the treatment area should be avoided.

71. The Organization for Safety and Asepsis Procedures (OSAP) identifies the classification of clinical touch surfaces to include which of the following?
   b. OSAP identifies light handles, dental unit controls, and chair switches as clinical touch surfaces. Many touch surfaces are identified in the other answers, but there is a distracter in each of these other answers that makes them inaccurate.

72. Which of the following is *not* an acceptable method of preventing surface contamination?
   b. The use of alcohol is not acceptable by any of the agencies that are concerned with dental office treatment areas.

73. What are standard precautions?
   c. Standard precautions referred to in the OSHA Bloodborne Pathogens Standard are based on the concept that all human blood and body fluids (including saliva) are to be treated as if known to be infected with bloodborne diseases.

74. The best time to clean and disinfect a dental prosthesis or impression that will be processed in the office laboratory is:
   d. A prosthesis should be cleaned as soon as possible after removal from a patient's mouth to avoid potential cross-contamination.

75. A victim who feels the effects of a chemical spill immediately, with symptoms of dizziness, headache, nausea, and vomiting, is experiencing:
   b. Acute chemical toxicity results from high levels of exposure over a short period. Acute toxicity is often caused by a chemical spill, in which the exposure is sudden and often involves a large amount of the chemical. The victim may feel the effects immediately and shown symptoms of dizziness, fainting, headache, nausea, and vomiting.

76. _____ is considered regulated waste and requires special disposal.
   a. Human tissue is considered pathologic waste and requires special handling and disposal. It is categorized as infectious waste, also called regulated waste or biohazardous waste. This category includes soft tissue, extracted teeth, blood, and blood-soaked materials as well as sharps.

77. Repeated exposure to chemicals at low levels for extended periods of time can result in liver disease or brain disorders that would be examples of:
   a. Chronic chemical toxicity results from many repeated exposures of lower levels, over a long period of time such as months or even years. The victim may experience many effects of chronic toxicity, such as liver disease, brain disorders, cancer, or infertility.

78. How often should the dental assistant or office safety supervisor check the contents of the emergency kit to determine that the contents are in place and within the expiration date?
    b. Because a variety of drugs may be kept in the emergency kit, many of which will have expiration dates, the emergency kit should be checked monthly.

79. The floor in the entry to the dental office was wet. A patient slipped on the floor during entry to the office. There was no signage to include a potential slippery floor. Which of the following would be *true*?
    a. The office owner, whether the dentist or another building owner, must post or place signs when potential dangerous situations exist, such as the wet floor. In this case, the building owner is responsible for the placement of the sign and for the training of persons who are responsible for placing such signage.

80. Wastes are classified as hazardous if they are:
    a. If a waste product is ignitable or flammable, it is considered to be hazardous according to the EPA.

81. All waste containers that hold potentially infectious materials must:
    b. Infectious waste (regulated waste) must be labeled with the universal biohazard symbol, identified in compliance with local regulations, or both. Once contaminated waste leaves the office, it is then regulated by the EPA and by state and local laws.

82. Scrap dental amalgam should be collected and stored in:
    a. Scrap dental amalgam is stored in a designated, dry, airtight container. It is considered hazardous waste and poses a risk to humans and to the environment.

83. Which government agency enforces the disposal of regulated waste?
    b. The EPA is responsible for regulated waste once it leaves the dental office.

84. The OSHA Hazard Communications Standard requires employers to do all *except* which of the following?
    d. The employer is required by the OSHA Hazard Communications Standard to accomplish all of the statements in a, b, and c. It is not required by this standard to have employees submit to an annual urinalysis test.

85. Each member of the dental staff is required to have available and know the location of which of the following item(s) in the event of a heart attack or closed or blocked airway?
    b. Each dental health care worker must know the location of the oxygen tank in case of emergencies. Periodic updates in emergency procedures should be offered to the staff.

86. Hazard communication training must include all of the following *except* _____.
    d. The waiver of hepatitis C vaccinations is not an appropriate response to hazard communication training for the dental staff. Each of the other tasks are required for the employer to make available for the staff.

87. A DHCW transfers a small amount of a glass ionomer cement into a smaller container for use on a patient at chairside. A new label must be placed on that container if:
    b. If the dental cement is not used up in its entirely by the end of the work shift, an appropriate label must be attached to the bottle to meet with the requirements of the Hazard Communication Standard issued by OSHA.

88. Hazard communication training must be provided:
    d. The Hazard Communication Standard issued by OSHA requires the dentist to provide hazard communication training to each employee and annually thereafter.

89. When recapping the needle, the dental assistant should use any of the following methods *except* _____.
    d. The dental assistant must never use a two-handed scoop method; it is potentially dangerous because the assistant could slip and cause a needle puncture.

90. Which of the following is *not* considered a "sharp"?
    b. The matrix retainer is not a sharp device. It is used to hold the matrix band, which is considered a sharp.

91. Which of the following is *not* a main concern as a microorganism in a dental unit water line?
    d. The first three microorganisms pose potential harmful infections under special conditions and in immunocompromised persons. *Lactobacillus* is not a microorganism of concern in the dental unit water line.

92. The ADA, OSAP, and CDC recommend that the dental assistant:
    b. Each of the above-mentioned organizations concur that flushing of the dental unit waterlines for 30 seconds each morning and between patients will promote safe practice. This can be followed up by flushing and cleaning at the end of the day.

93. Shortly after donning the required PPE, the dental health care worker notices the following symptoms: watering eyes, nasal congestion, sneezing, coughing, wheezing, shortness of breath, and even dizziness. This person may be experiencing which type of reaction?
    a. Because this condition occurred immediately upon donning the PPEs, the reaction can be identified as an immediate hypersensitivity. A reaction like this generally occurs within 20 minutes.

94. Which of the following are the recommended five parts of the Hazard Communication Standard?
    b. According to the Hazard Communication Standard of OSHA, the five basic components include a written program, inventory of hazardous chemicals, MSDS for every chemical, proper labeling of containers, and employee training.

95. Which of the following statements is *not* true?
    c. HIV is transmitted primarily from an infected person through the following routes: intimate sexual contact, exposure to blood, blood-contaminated body fluids or blood products, or perinatal contact.

96. Switching to instruments with large, round diameters and contra-angled shanks may _____ the symptoms associated with carpal tunnel syndrome.
    a. By modifying the size and design of the instruments used at chairside, it may be possible to reduce the symptoms of carpal tunnel syndrome.

97. Which of these factors should *not* be practiced during the use of nitrous oxide during conscious sedation?
    a. During the use of nitrous oxide, you should avoid having a conversation with the patient as this will cause movement of the nasal mask and cause potential gas leaks around the mask.

98. Distillation of water is a _____ process that may remove volatile chemicals, endotoxins, and some microorganisms.
    c. The use of distilled water may ensure the elimination of volatile chemicals, endotoxins and some microorganisms, thus potentially providing a safer water for dental office use.

99. Which of the following statements is *not* true regarding the use of biohazard warning labels?
    d. White or green bags are not compliant in meeting the OSHA Standard for biohazard labeling.

100. OSHA requires the use of standard precautions for _____.
    d. OSHA requires that standard precautions be used for all patients. Therefore blood and other body fluids from all patients are treated as potentially infections.

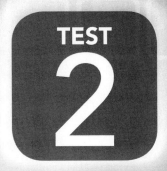

General Chairside, Radiation Health and Safety, and Infection Control

General Chairside

Directions: Select the response that best answers each of the following questions. Only one response is correct.

1. A patient displaying hypertension would have a blood pressure of about:
   a. 80/110 mm Hg
   b. 120/80 mm Hg
   c. 130/64 mm Hg
   d. 180/96 mm Hg

2. A patient presents appearing "flushed" and states that he has an infection. Which temperature would most likely be measured?
   a. 92° F
   b. 97.8° F
   c. 99.6° F
   d. 102° F

3. The normal blood pressure classification for adults is:
   a. 100/50 mm Hg
   b. 120/80 mm Hg
   c. 140/95 mm Hg
   d. 160/110 mm Hg

4. The most common site for taking a patient's pulse when performing cardiopulmonary resuscitation is the:
   a. brachial artery
   b. carotid artery
   c. radial artery
   d. femoral artery

5. Consent is:
   a. an involuntary act
   b. voluntary acceptance or agreement to what is planned or done by another person
   c. only necessary for surgical procedures
   d. something that any person over 21 may give for another's treatment

6. Using Black's classification of cavities, a pit lesion on the buccal surface of molars and premolars is considered a Class _____ restoration or cavity.
   a. I
   b. II
   c. III
   d. V

7. The abbreviation used in the progress notes or chart to indicate a mesioocclusodistal lesion would be:
   a. MeOcDi
   b. DOM
   c. MOD
   d. MOB

8. The tooth-numbering system that gives each of the four quadrants its own tooth bracket made up of a vertical and horizontal line is referred to as the:
   a. Universal System
   b. Palmer Notation System
   c. Fédération Dentaire Internationale System
   d. Bracket Numbering System

9. Any tooth that remains unerupted in the jaw beyond the time at which it should normally erupt is referred to as being:
   a. abraded
   b. impacted
   c. ankylosed
   d. fused

10. A tray is set up from _____ to _____.
    a. left to right
    b. right to left
    c. top to bottom

11. The "A" in the ABCDs of basic life support stands for:
    a. access
    b. automatic
    c. airway
    d. assess

12. An arrow used as a charting symbol indicates which of the following?
    a. tooth is mobile
    b. tooth has drifted
    c. tooth is missing
    d. tooth has a crown

13. A periodontal probe is an example of which type of instrument?
    a. examination
    b. hand cutting
    c. restorative
    d. accessory

14. A patient, aged 78, presents for a partial denture examination. She appears to weigh about 100 lbs, is frail, has a rather slow gait, and indicates she has no health contraindications, is only taking some vitamins, but does have some slight hearing problems. When her blood pressure is taken, it is likely to be:
    a. 106/52 mm Hg
    b. 52/106 mm Hg
    c. 190/90 mm Hg
    d. 210/112 mm Hg

15. The normal pulse rate for a resting adult is:
    a. 35 to 50 beats per minute
    b. 50 to 90 beats per minute
    c. 60 to 100 beats per minute
    d. 70 to 120 beats per minute

16. A new patient tells you that her blood pressure normally is low. If this is true, her blood pressure could be which of the following?
    a. 100/50 mm Hg
    b. 120/80 mm Hg
    c. 140/95 mm Hg
    d. 160/110 mm Hg

17. A patient displaying hypertension would have a blood pressure of about:
    a. 80/110 mm Hg
    b. 120/80 mm Hg
    c. 130/64 mm Hg
    d. 180/96 mm Hg

18. A patient with hypothermia would have a temperature of:
    a. 90° F
    b. 97.8° F
    c. 99.6° F
    d. 102° F

19. The automated external defibrillator (AED) is used for all *except* to _____.
    a. reestablish the proper heart rhythm by defibrillation
    b. automatically perform CPR for 15 minutes
    c. shock the heart
    d. monitor the patient's heart rhythm

20. _____ can be life threatening and is indicated by nausea and vomiting, shortness of breath, and loss of consciousness.
    a. Anaphylaxis
    b. Syncope
    c. Low blood glucose
    d. High blood pressure

21. The respirations of a patient who is hyperventilating will be exemplified by:
    a. slow respiration rate
    b. excessively short, rapid breaths
    c. excessively long, rapid breaths
    d. gurgling

22. The respiration pattern of a patient in a state of tachypnea has:
    a. a slow respiration rate
    b. excessively short, rapid breaths
    c. excessively long, rapid breaths
    d. a gurgling sound

Review the figure below to answer questions 23 through 27.

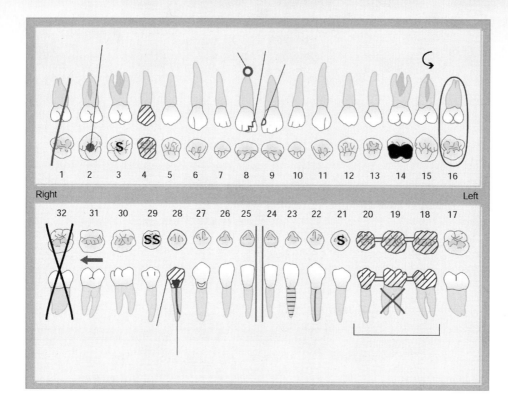

23. The symbol on tooth No. 31 indicates it is:
   a. mobile
   b. drifted distally
   c. drifted mesially
   d. rotated

24. The symbol on tooth No. 8 indicates it will need to have:
   a. periodontal treatment and then a restoration to replace the distoincisal angle
   b. endodontic treatment and then a restoration to replace the mesioincisal angle
   c. periodontal treatment and then a restoration to replace the incisal edge
   d. endodontic treatment and then a restoration to replace the distoincisal angle

25. The symbol between teeth No. 24 and No. 25 indicates:
   a. a supernumerary tooth present
   b. a displaced frenum attachment
   c. heavy calculus
   d. a diastema is present

26. The symbol on tooth No. 23 indicates that this tooth:
   a. has a fractured root
   b. is an implant
   c. has a root canal
   d. has a post and core

27. The symbol on tooth No. 3 indicates that this tooth:
   a. has sealant placed
   b. has a stainless steel crown
   c. needs to have a sealant
   d. has occlusal staining

Review the figure below to answer questions 28 and 29.

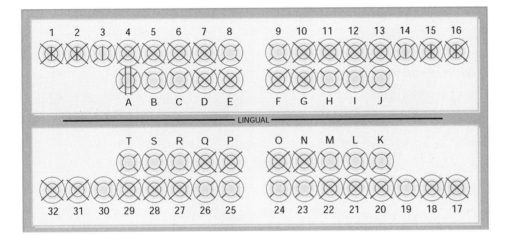

28. How many permanent teeth have erupted?
   a. 6
   b. 10
   c. 12
   d. 14

29. How many permanent teeth are present on the mandible?
   a. 6
   b. 10
   c. 12
   d. 14

30. The examination technique in which the examiner uses his or her fingers and hands to feel for size, texture, and consistency of hard and soft tissue is called:
   a. detection
   b. palpation
   c. probing
   d. extraoral examination

31. Which of the following statements is *not* true as it relates to a patient's respiration?
   a. If a patient knows the breaths are being monitored, he or she will usually change his or her breathing pattern.
   b. For children and teenagers, the respiration rate is higher than that of an adult.
   c. A person's respirations normally are not noticeable unless the person is having trouble taking a breath.
   d. Respirations are normally higher in count per minute than the pulse rate.

32. Most local anesthetic agents used for dental procedures are:
   a. short-acting
   b. intermediate-acting
   c. long-acting

33. In the United States, nitrous oxide gas lines are color-coded _____ and oxygen lines are color-coded _____.
   a. red, blue
   b. green, blue
   c. blue, red
   d. blue, green

34. The dental assistant's responsibility in an emergency situation is to:
   a. recognize the symptoms and signs of a significant medical complaint
   b. provide appropriate support in implementing emergency procedures
   c. diagnose a specific condition or emergency situation
   d. both a and b

35. A condition called _____ will result if an alginate impression absorbs additional water by being stored in water or in a very wet paper towel.
   a. syneresis
   b. hydrocolloid
   c. imbibition
   d. polymerization

36. A patient who displays symptoms of intermittent blinking, mouth movements, blank stare, and nonresponsiveness to surroundings may be displaying symptoms of:
   a. petit mal seizure
   b. grand mal seizure
   c. hypoglycemia
   d. hyperglycemia

37. The water-to-powder ratio generally used for an adult mandibular impression is _____ measures of water, _____ scoops of powder.
   a. 3, 3
   b. 4, 3
   c. 2, 4
   d. 2, 2

38. The RDAs are the levels of essential nutrients that are needed by individuals on a daily basis. RDA stands for:
   a. recommended dietary allowance
   b. regulated daily amount
   c. regular daily amount
   d. recommended daily allowance

39. The only nutrients that can build and repair body tissues are:
   a. proteins
   b. fats
   c. carbohydrates
   d. minerals

40. _____ can prevent cholesterol from oxidizing and damaging arteries.
   a. Vitamins
   b. Minerals
   c. Lipids
   d. Antioxidants

41. The retromolar area is reproduced in the _____ impression.
   a. maxillary
   b. mandibular

42. Which of the following instruments would be used to measure the depth of the gingival sulcus?
   a. periodontal probe
   b. cowhorn explorer
   c. right angle explorer
   d. shepherd's hook

43. Which of the following instruments has sharp, round, angular tips used to detect tooth anomalies?
   a. periodontal probe
   b. cowhorn explorer
   c. right angle explorer
   d. shepherd's hook explorer

44. Which instrument is commonly used to scale surfaces in the anterior region of the mouth?
   a. curet scaler
   b. Gracey scaler
   c. straight sickle scaler
   d. modified sickle scaler

45. Which instrument is used to scale deep periodontal pockets or furcation areas?
   a. curet scaler
   b. Gracey scaler
   c. straight sickle scaler
   d. modified sickle scaler

46. In the drawing below, which area stabilizes the clamp to the tooth.

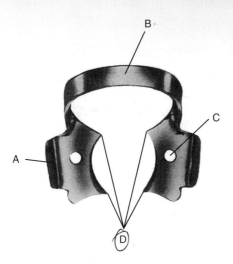

47. When the operator is working in the labial of tooth No. 9, the HVE tip is held:
  a. on the labial surface of the tooth being prepared
  b. on the opposite side of the tooth being prepared
  c. in the retromolar area
  d. in the vestibule

48. A right-handed dentist is doing a preparation on 30MO. The dental assistant places the HVE tip:
  a. on the buccal of No. 30
  b. on the buccal of No. 19
  c. on the lingual of No. 30
  d. on the occlusal of No. 31

49. The angle of the bevel of the HVE tip should always be:
  a. parallel to the buccal or lingual surfaces
  b. at right angles to the buccal and lingual surfaces
  c. parallel to the occlusal surface
  d. in whatever position the assistant is comfortable

50. Which of the following is a thermoplastic material used to stabilize an anterior clamp?
  a. driangle
  b. floss
  c. dental compound
  d. sticky wax

51. The wooden wedge is placed in the gingival embrasure area for Class II restorations to accomplish all *except* which of the following?
  a. provide a missing proximal wall
  b. adapt the band to the cervical margin
  c. aid in preventing overhangs
  d. maintain proximal contact

52. Which of the following techniques could be used for caries removal?
    a. No. 2 RA bur and enamel hatchet
    b. No. 1/4 FG and spoon excavator
    c. No. 2 RA and spoon excavator
    d. No. 1/4 FG and explorer

53. Select the instrument that will be used to carve the distal surface of an amalgam restoration placed on 30DO.

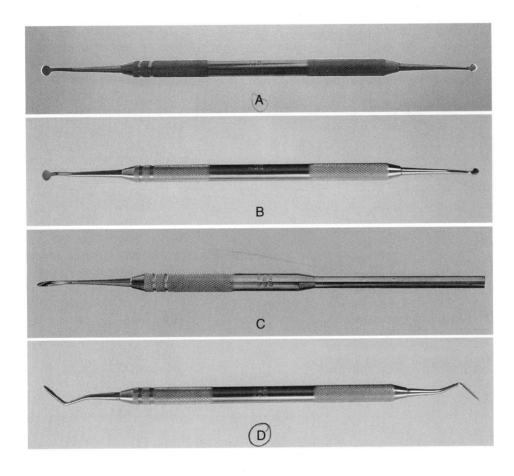

A

B

C

D

54. From the photograph below, select the instrument that would be used to attach to the rubber dam clamps.

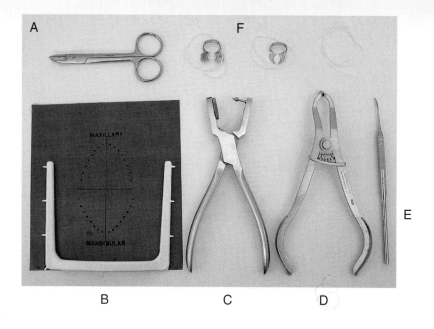

55. Which of the following instruments is a Hedstrom file?

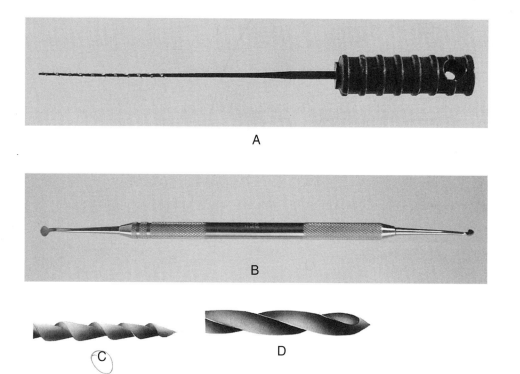

56. Which of the photographs below illustrates an orthodontic hemostat?

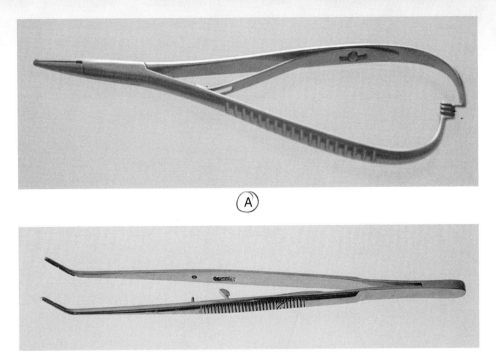

Ⓐ

B

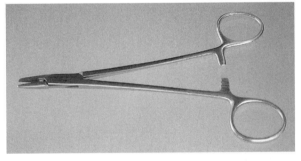

C

57. Which instrument would be used to check for an overhang on a newly placed restoration?
   a. spoon excavator
   b. Ward's carver
   c. Hollenback carver
   d. explorer

58. Which of the following instruments would be the least likely to be used for placing a cavity liner?
  a. spoon excavator
  b. explorer
  c. ball burnisher
  d. amalgam condenser

59. Under which of the following conditions would the shade for an anterior esthetic restoration *not* be selected?
  a. with natural light and moist environment
  b. after cavity preparation and medication
  c. before application of rubber dam
  d. within the same oral environment as the tooth being restored

60. At what time can the final polish of a light-cured composite be accomplished?
  a. within 10 minutes
  b. within 20 to 30 minutes
  c. after 8 hours
  d. as soon as the material is polymerized

61. Which of the following would *not* be used for smooth surface carving in an amalgam procedure?
  a. Hollenback carver
  b. Ward's C carver
  c. cleoid discoid carver

62. Which of the following endodontic instruments is used to curette the inside of the tooth to the base of the pulp chamber?
  a. long-shank spoon
  b. reamer
  c. file
  d. explorer

63. Using the operating zones based on the "clock concept," the assistant's zone for a right-handed operator is:
  a. 2 to 4 o'clock
  b. 12 to 2 o'clock
  c. 10 to 12 o'clock
  d. 8 to 10 o'clock

64. A finger rest that stabilizes the hand so that there is less possibility of slipping or traumatizing the tissue in the mouth is known as a _____.
  a. hinge point
  b. rest point
  c. fulcrum
  d. base

65. Which of the following types of anesthesia produce a state of unconsciousness?
    a. local
    b. conscious sedation
    c. inhalation
    d. general

66. A cotton roll remains attached to the buccal mucosa after treatment has been completed. The safest way to remove the cotton roll is to:
    a. pull it away from the tissue quickly
    b. moisten it and then remove it
    c. ask the patient to gently remove it
    d. apply pressure to the site and then remove it

67. The time from when the local anesthetic takes complete effect until the complete reversal of anesthesia is the _____ of the anesthetic agent.
    a. duration
    b. induction
    c. innervation
    d. compression

68. The lengths of the needles used in dentistry for local anesthesia administration are:
    a. 1½ and 2 inches
    b. 1 and 1⅜ inches
    c. ½ and 1½ inches
    d. ⅝ and 1 inch

69. The stage of anesthesia when the patient passes through excitement and becomes calm, feels no pain or sensation, and soon becomes unconscious is referred to as stage ____ of anesthesia.
    a. I
    b. II
    c. III
    d. IV

70. The most common type of attachment for fixed orthodontic appliances is the:
    a. orthodontic band
    b. bonded bracket
    c. arch wire
    d. separator

71. When a health contraindication is present that prevents the use of a vasoconstrictor, the retraction cord is impregnated with _____ and the cord may have a _____ agent applied to it to control bleeding.
    a. epinephrine, hemostatic
    b. aluminum chloride, galvanic
    c. sodium chloride, galvanic
    d. aluminum chloride, hemostatic

72. The procedural tray shown below is used to:
   a. place separators
   b. fit and cement orthodontic bands
   c. direct bond orthodontic bands
   d. place and remove ligature ties

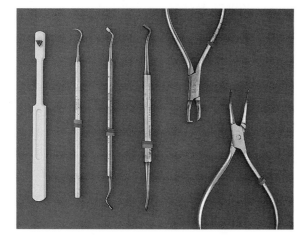

73. The instruments shown below from left to right are:
   a. three-pronged pliers, posterior band remover, ligature pin
   b. wire bending pliers, Howe pliers, Weingart utility pliers
   c. bird beak pliers, contouring pliers, Weingart utility pliers

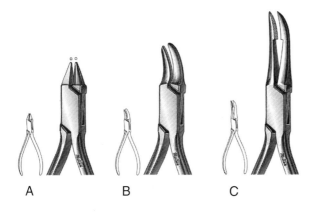

A   B   C

74. A nonsurgical technique that uses a sterile flat-ended brush to gather the surface cells from a suspect oral lesion is a(n) _____ biopsy.
   a. incisional
   b. excisional
   c. exfoliative
   d. clinical

75. The scalpel blade that resembles a bird's beak is a:
   a. No. 11
   b. No. 12
   c. No. 14
   d. No. 15

76. The ideal candidate for dental implants meets which of the following criteria?
   a. has good health and adequate alveolar bone
   b. is willing to commit to conscientious oral hygiene and regular dental visits
   c. is concerned about the financial investment of implants
   d. both a and b

77. Which tissues are those that surround the root of the tooth?
   a. periradicular
   b. periapical
   c. gingival
   d. osseous

78. The process of removing bacteria, necrotic tissue, and organic debris from the root canal is called:
   a. opening the canal
   b. obturating the canal
   c. debriding the canal
   d. shaping the canal

79. From the photograph below, which instrument is a K-type file?

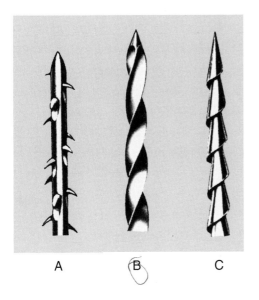

A   B   C

80. Which of the following is *not* a surgical procedure performed to remove defects or restore normal contours to the bone?
   a. osseous surgery
   b. oteoplasty
   c. osteoectomy
   d. gingivoplasty

81. _____ is a small rubber, silicone, or plastic device that is slid onto an endodontic instrument to prevent perforation of the apex during instrumentation.
    a. Glide
    b. Separator
    c. Stop
    d. Ring

82. A dentist with a license in the specialty of dentistry that is involved in the diagnosis and treatment of the supporting tissues of the teeth is a(n) _____.
    a. endodontist
    b. periodontist
    c. orthodontist
    d. prosthodontist

83. A condition of periodontal disease when the gingival tissues migrate away from the tooth, leaving portions of the roots of the teeth exposed below the cementoenamel junction, is called _____ _____.
    a. bruxism
    b. gingival recession
    c. alveolitis
    d. occlusal trauma

84. Vertical bitewing radiographs are especially valuable in periodontics to determine the _____.
    a. amount of decay
    b. location of decay
    c. bone height
    d. extent of crestal bone loss

85. Indications for use of an ultrasonic scaler include all of the following *except* _____:
    a. removal of supragingival calculus and difficult stain
    b. cleaning of furcation areas
    c. removal of orthodontic cements, or debonding
    d. cardiac pacemaker

86. Which of the following is *not* an advantage of laser surgery in periodontics?
    a. hemostasis
    b. risk of bloodborne contamination reduced
    c. swelling and scarring reduced
    d. elimination of any pain or discomfort

87. A double-ended knife with kidney-shaped blades commonly used in periodontal surgery is known as a(n):
    a. Orban knife
    b. Kirkland knife
    c. No. 12 blade
    d. No. 15 blade

88. In which of the following procedures could the patient be placed in an upright position?
    a. composite procedure
    b. removal of a posterior tooth
    c. polishing the teeth after a prophylaxis
    d. taking diagnostic impressions

Review the figure below to answer questions 89 and 90.

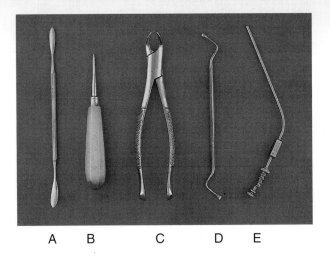

A   B   C   D   E

89. Select the straight elevator. b

90. Which instrument would be used to debride the interior of the tooth socket after an extraction? 1

91. A patient is to take a medication three times a day. The prescription will indicate to the pharmacy that it is taken:
 a. BID
 b. TID
 c. QID
 d. q.d.

92. If the signature line on a prescription states *1 tab QID prn pain*, it indicates that the patient would take the medication:
 a. one tablet daily as needed
 b. one tablet every 4 hours for pain
 c. one tablet four times a day as needed for pain
 d. one tablet for 4 days

93. An antibiotic _____.
 a. reduces anxiety and tension
 b. slows the clotting of blood
 c. kills or inhibits the growth of microorganisms
 d. reduces the level of pain

94. An example of an anticoagulant is _____.
 a. Ceclor
 b. Librium
 c. Prozac
 d. Coumadin

95. Which is the correct sequence for placing sealants?
   a. etch, isolate, clean
   b. isolate, clean, etch
   c. clean, isolate, etch

96. The type of implant used primarily on patients with severely resorbed ridges, and only if there is no other options is _____.
   a. transosteal
   b. endosteal
   c. subperiosteal

97. Addition of very warm water to an alginate mix will cause the setting time to be:
   a. increased
   b. decreased

98. A negative reproduction of the patient's dental arch is referred to as a(n):
   a. die
   b. model
   c. cast
   d. impression

99. The impression automix system can be used for all but which of the following?
   a. syringe material
   b. tray material
   c. bite registration
   d. putty wash

100. The process by which the resin material is changed from a pliable state to a hardened restoration is known as:
   a. light curing
   b. exothermic curing
   c. microcuring
   d. macrocuring

101. If humidity is high while mixing a final impression material, the setting time may be:
   a. decreased
   b. increased

102. Select two terms that describe the purpose and consistency of a dental cement used for the seating of a temporary crown.
   a. base and secondary consistency
   b. cementation and secondary consistency
   c. base and primary consistency
   d. cementation and primary consistency

103. An onlay is a cast restoration that differs from an inlay in that the onlay includes the _____, _____, and some or all of the _____ to avoid future fracture.
   a. complete occlusal table, both proximal surfaces, cusp surfaces
   b. occlusal table, one proximal surface, buccal and lingial surfaces
   c. one proximal surface, buccal surfaces, lingual surfaces
   d. buccal or lingual surface, two proximal surfaces, occlusal table

104. A resin bonded bridge is commonly referred to as a _____.
   a. traditional bridge
   b. Maryland bridge
   c. temporary bridge
   d. Wisconsin bridge

105. When surgical retraction is performed rather than using chemical gingival retraction, the procedure is referred to as _____.
   a. cold steel surgery
   b. electrosurgery
   c. electrolysis
   d. gingivectomy

106. Which of the following instruments is used to trim soft tissue during an oral surgery procedure?
   a. surgical curette
   b. suture scissors
   c. surgical scissors
   d. scalpel

107. The eating disorder that can easily be recognized in the dental office by severe wear on the lingual surface of the teeth caused by stomach acid from repeated vomiting is:
   a. bulimia
   b. binge eating
   c. anorexia nervosa
   d. female athlete triathlon

108. Inflammation of the supporting tissues of the teeth that begins with _____ can progress into the connective tissue and alveolar bone that supports the teeth and become _____.
   a. gingivitis, glossitis
   b. periodontitis, gingivitis
   c. gingivitis, periodontitis
   d. gingivitis, gangrene

109. The dentist retires to another state and closes the practice. The entire staff is released from employment and the records remain in the office, but the patients are not notified of the dentist's retirement. Failure to notify the patients of the changes in the practice is called:
   a. assault
   b. abandonment
   c. malpractice
   d. noncompliance

110. The MyPyramid, formerly known as the Food Guide Pyramid, is an outline of what to eat each day. The food group represented by the second smallest section on the pyramid is:
   a. dairy
   b. meat and beans
   c. oils
   d. vegetables

111. _____ are found mainly in fruits, grains, and vegetables and _____ are found in processed foods such as jelly, bread, crackers, and cookies.
   a. Proteins, carbohydrates
   b. Complex carbohydrates, fats
   c. Complex carbohydrates, simple sugars
   d. Proteins, simple sugars

112. The patient's record indicates that the status of the gingival tissue is bulbous, flattened, punched-out, and cratered. This statement describes:
   a. gingival color
   b. gingival contour
   c. consistency of the gingival
   d. surface texture of the gingival

113. Supragingival calculus is found on the _____ of the teeth, above the margin of the _____.
   a. cervical region, periodontal ligament
   b. clinical crowns, gingiva
   c. anatomical crowns, periodontal ligament
   d. cervical margins, apex

114. Subgingival calculus occurs _____ the gingival margin and can be _____ in color due to subgingival bleeding.
   a. above, yellow
   b. below, yellow
   c. above, red
   d. below, black

115. Which are examples of local risk factors for periodontal disease?
   a. oral hygiene, osteoporosis, smoking
   b. overhanging restorations, orthodontic appliances, removable partial dentures
   c. stress, HIV/AIDS, osteoporosis, diabetes
   d. poor oral hygiene, stress, medications, smoking, diabetes

116. Which of the following is *not* a component of a clinical record?
   a. clinical chart
   b. health history
   c. medical history
   d. recall card

117. Which of the following records is considered a vital record?
   a. patient clinical chart
   b. bank reconciliation
   c. petty cash voucher
   d. cancelled check

118. Which member of the dental team is legally required to report suspected child abuse?
   a. all members
   b. dentist
   c. dental assistant
   d. dental hygienist

119. The dentist informs you that a patient will need three appointments to complete a three–unit bridge. These appointments will likely be to:
  a. prepare the teeth, try on the bridge components, and seat the bridge
  b. take diagnostic models, prepare the teeth, and seat the temporary/provisional crown
  c. prepare the teeth, take the impressions, and seat the bridge

120. The administrative assistant has failed to maintain the recall system for the past four months. Which is likely to occur?
  a. there will be evidence of decreased productivity
  b. the patients will not mind
  c. there will be more time to work on incomplete projects

Radiation Health and Safety

Directions: Select the response that best answers each of the following questions. Only one response is correct.

1. Label the solutions used in an automatic film processor from left to right.
   a. water wash, developing solution, fixing solution
   b. developing solution, fixing solution, water wash
   c. fixing solution, developing solution, water wash

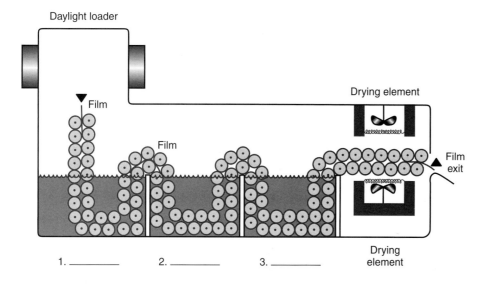

2. What is the landmark indicated by the arrows?
   a. mental foramen
   b. incisive foramen
   c. cervical spine
   d. genial tubercles

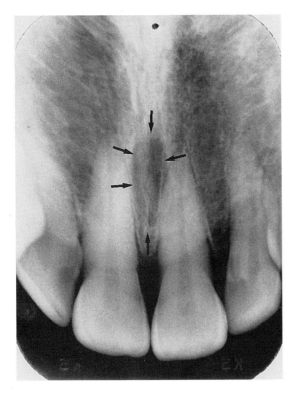

3. What is the landmark circled on the radiograph?
   a. mental foramen
   b. lingual foramen
   c. mandibular canal
   d. genial tubercles

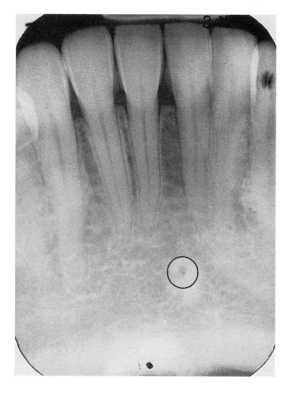

4. A bitewing film shows the _____ of both the _____ and _____.
   a. entire tooth, maxilla, mandible
   b. crowns, right, left
   c. crowns, maxilla, mandible
   d. entire tooth, posterior, anterior

5. _____ is an example of a patient protection technique used before x-ray exposure.
   a. Proper film processing
   b. Proper prescribing of radiographs
   c. A lead apron
   d. A thyroid collar

6. Which of the following is the recommended size of the beam at the patient's face?
   a. 2.75 inches
   b. 3.25 inches
   c. 3.50 inches
   d. 4 inches

7. The _____ is an extension of the x-ray tubehead and is used to direct the x-ray beam.
   a. aluminum disk
   b. PID (position indicating devices)
   c. collimator
   d. filter

8. The collimator:
   a. is always round
   b. restricts the size and shape of the x-ray beam
   c. is a solid piece of aluminum
   d. is fitted within the copper stem beneath the molybdenum cup

9. Which of the following types of PIDs do *not* produce scatter radiation?
   a. rectangular
   b. round
   c. conical
   d. both a and b

10. The thyroid collar:
   a. is recommended for all intraoral films
   b. is recommended for all extraoral films
   c. may exist as a separate shield or as part of the lead apron
   d. both a and c

11. After the lead apron is used it should be:
   a. disinfected
   b. folded and stored
   c. hung up or laid on a rounded bar
   d. both a and c

12. The_____ film provides a wide view of the maxilla and mandible.
   a. bitewing
   b. periapical
   c. panoramic
   d. cephalometric

13. _____ film can be used in cassettes.
   a. Intensifying
   b. Panoramic
   c. Extraoral
   d. Intraoral

14. Which device is used to assist in the position of the PID in relation to the tooth and film?
   a. film holder
   b. bite blocks
   c. beam alignment device
   d. cotton rolls

15. Rules of radiation protection for the operator include all of the following *except* _____.
   a. never stand in the direct line of the primary beam
   b. always stand behind a lead barrier or a proper thickness of drywall
   c. never stand closer than 3 feet from the x-ray unit during an exposure
   d. monitor radiation exposure

16. In order to increase the contrast on a radiograph, one should _____ the kilovoltage peak.
   a. decrease
   b. increase

17. Which of the following statements is *true* about duplicating films?
   a. The duplicated films always remain in the dental office, and the originals are transferred.
   b. Duplicating film does not need safelight conditions.
   c. The duplicating film has emulsion on both sides.
   d. If more film density is needed, the exposure time is shortened.

18. Radiation caries is most often seen on teeth:
   a. interproximally
   b. on occlusal surfaces
   c. at the cervical line circumferentially
   d. around crowns

19. A tissue that lies within the primary dental beam and is very radiosensitive is the _____.
   a. tongue
   b. cornea
   c. thyroid
   d. inner ear

20. When x-ray exposure time is increased, there is _____ density of the radiograph.
   a. increased
   b. decreased

21. The overall blackness or darkness of a film is _____.
   a. contrast
   b. density
   c. quality
   d. intensity

22. Which of these would appear radiopaque on a radiograph?
   a. tooth decay
   b. dental pulp
   c. tooth enamel
   d. abscesses

23. If the radiographic processing time is too long, the film will appear _____.
   a. dark
   b. light
   c. clear
   d. fogged

24. The hardening agent in processing fixer is(are):
 a. elon and hydroquinone
 b. sodium sulfite
 c. potassium alum
 d. acetic acid and sulfuric acid

25. Failure to add replenisher as needed each day to an automatic processor will result in:
 a. overexposed film
 b. poor-quality films
 c. underexposed film
 d. clear films

26. X-ray film can be removed from the fixer after _____ minutes for a wet reading and _____.
 a. 7 minutes, then air dried
 b. 3 minutes, returned to fixer for the remainder of processing
 c. 5 minutes, returned to fixer for the remainder of processing
 d. 12 minutes, then air dried

27. What is the optimum development time and temperature for radiographic films using manual processing?
 a. 72 degrees for 5 minutes
 b. 68 degrees for 12 minutes
 c. 78 degrees for 12 minutes
 d. 68 degrees for 5 minutes

28. An overdeveloped film may be caused by which of the following?
 a. inadequate development time
 b. solution that is too cool
 c. excessive development time
 d. depleted developer solution

29. In a dental practice where many HIV-positive patients are treated, the film rollers in the automatic processor should be:
 a. scrubbed with an abrasive cleaner every day
 b. autoclaved every day
 c. disinfected after every use
 d. treated in the usual accepted manner

30. When using the bisecting technique, the imaginary angle that is bisected is formed between the long axis of the tooth and the:
 a. long axis of the PID
 b. horizontal axis of the film
 c. long axis of the film
 d. horizontal axis of the tubehead

31. For patients with bilateral mandibular impactions, the right and left lateral oblique techniques have been replaced by:
 a. occlusal films
 b. posterior anterior projections
 c. panoramic films
 d. double periapicals

32. In TMJ radiography, it is preferable to take films in the _____ position(s).
a. open only
b. closed only
c. open and closed
d. partially opened

33. The computer used for digital imaging:
a. cannot be used for other office functions
b. can be used for other office functions
c. is the most expensive component of the system
d. is nonessential hardware

34. What is the problem with this radiograph?
a. overdeveloped
b. developer cutoff
c. reticulation
d. static marks

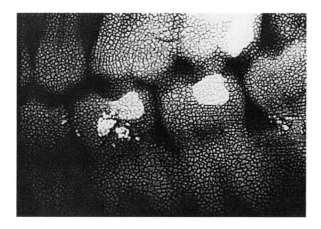

35. On intraoral radiographs, when the patient's right is on your right, this is called _____ mounting.
a. labial
b. neutral
c. cross
d. lingual

36. A periapical lesion would appear _____ on processed radiographs.
a. radiopaque
b. radiolucent
c. geometric
d. poorly defined

37. Radiographically, the appearance of a "dry socket" resembles:
a. normal healing socket
b. osteomyelitis
c. infection
d. a cyst

38. Personnel monitoring of radiation exposure:
   a. identifies the location of exposure to primary beams
   b. identifies occupational exposure to radiation
   c. measures the amount of exposure for each patient
   d. alerts the operator when the maximum amount of exposure for the month has been reached

39. When a patient expresses concern about the need for radiographs, which of the following statements should be avoided?
   a. "The doctor orders radiographs based on your individual needs."
   b. "We use a lead apron and thyroid collar to protect your body from stray radiation."
   c. "We use high-speed film that requires only minimal amounts of radiation."
   d. "It is routine in this office according to the doctor's orders."

40. The _____ radiograph provides a view that shows the tooth crown, root tip, and surrounding structures of a specific area.
   a. bitewing
   b. periapical
   c. panoramic
   d. cephalometric

41. Which type of PID would be most effective in reducing patient exposure?
   a. conical
   b. 16-inch round PID
   c. 8-inch rectangular PID
   d. 16-inch rectangular PID

42. Which of the following conditions exist on this film?
   a. a fixed bridge between the second premolar and second molar
   b. open contacts between maxillary premolars
   c. open contacts between the molars
   d. pulp stone on the second molar

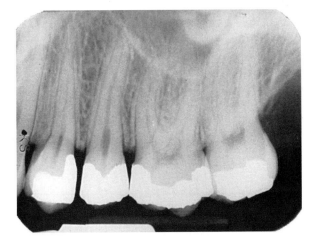

43. What is the landmark indicated by the arrows?
- **a.** mental foramen
- **b.** lingual foramen
- **c.** mandibular canal
- **d.** genial tubercles

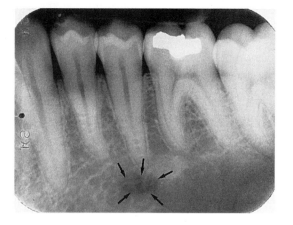

44. What is the landmark indicated by the arrows?
- **a.** coronoid process
- **b.** condyle
- **c.** internal oblique ridge
- **d.** mandibular canal

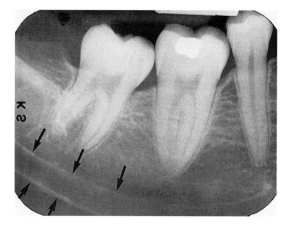

45. What is the landmark indicated by the arrows?
   a. zygomatic process of the maxilla
   b. floor of the frontal sinus
   c. floor of the maxillary sinus
   d. zygomatic arch

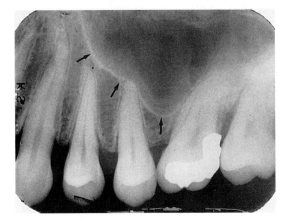

46. A _____ is defined as a marked prominence or projection of bone.
   a. ridge
   b. spine
   c. process
   d. foramen

47. The sensitivity of a film to radiation exposure is _____.
   a. film size
   b. film speed
   c. film type
   d. film factor

48. Inherent filtration in the dental x-ray tubehead:
   a. includes filtration that takes place when the primary beam passes through the glass window of the x-ray tube, the insulating oil, and the tubehead seal
   b. includes the placement of aluminum disks in the path of the x-ray beam between the collimator and the tubehead seal
   c. alone meets the standards regulated by state and federal law
   d. is equivalent to approximately 5.0 mm of aluminum

49. Which is *not* one of the three basic types of PIDs?
   a. conical
   b. rectangular
   c. round
   d. square

50. At what age should a full adult series be considered for a child?
   a. 12 years
   b. 15 years.
   c. 9 years
   d. 7 years

51. The _____ radiographic view shows the crowns of teeth of both arches on one film.
   a. bitewing
   b. periapical
   c. panoramic
   d. cephalometric

52. Commercially available barrier envelopes:
   a. minimize contamination before exposure of the film
   b. minimize contamination after exposure of the film
   c. are made of a material that blocks the passage of photons
   d. are made of a material that blocks the passage of electrons

53. Occlusal film is so named because it is _____ than periapical or bitewing film and the patient _____ the entire film.
   a. smaller, occludes
   b. larger, occludes
   c. smaller, holds
   d. larger, holds

54. Exposed films should _____ dried and then placed in a _____ for transport to the darkroom for processing.
   a. not be, gloved hand
   b. be, gloved hand
   c. not be, disposable container
   d. be, disposable container

55. The _____ radiograph is the film of choice for the evaluation of apical lesions.
   a. occlusal
   b. periapical
   c. bitewing
   d. cephalograph

56. The radiograph most commonly exposed for an orthodontic patient is the:
   a. FMS
   b. panoramic
   c. cephalometric
   d. bitewing

57. The minimum number of exposures for a full mouth survey of radiographs would be:
   a. 8
   b. 14
   c. 18
   d. 24

58. Developer solution has a(n) _____ pH, and fixer solution has a(n) _____ pH.
    a. acidic, acidic
    b. acidic, basic
    c. basic, acidic
    d. basic, basic

59. The purpose of a hardening agent is to harden and shrink the:
    a. exposed silver halide crystals
    b. plastic film base
    c. unexposed silver halide crystals
    d. gelatin in the film emulsion

60. The purpose of the fixing agent is to remove all _____ from the film emulsion.
    a. unexposed silver halide crystals
    b. exposed silver halide crystals
    c. unexposed and exposed silver halide crystals
    d. of the emulsion

61. The film emulsion is hardened during which of the following stages of the development process?
    a. developing
    b. rinsing
    c. fixing
    d. washing

62. A stepwedge will reveal that radiographs taken at a higher kilovoltage peak will have _____ versus radiographs taken at a lower kilovoltage peak.
    a. long-scale contrast
    b. high contrast
    c. low contrast
    d. multiple areas of black and white

63. A radiograph that has _____ is said to have low contrast.
    a. a very dark overall appearance
    b. a very light overall appearance
    c. many shades of gray
    d. very dark areas and very light areas

64. Which of the following would appear the most radiolucent on a radiograph?
    a. composite
    b. amalgam
    c. pulp
    d. enamel

65. Which of the following would appear most radiopaque?
    a. composite
    b. amalgam
    c. pulp
    d. enamel

66. Label the orientation planes; sagittal, coronal, transverse

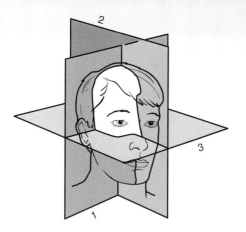

67. What is the landmark indicated by the arrows?
- **a.** mandibular canal
- **b.** lingual foramen
- **c.** internal oblique ridge
- **d.** mylohyoid ridge

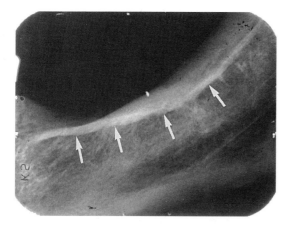

68. What is the landmark indicated by the arrows?
   a. pulp stone
   b. pulp cavity
   c. dentin
   d. cyst

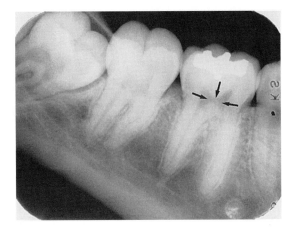

69. In this panoramic radiograph, which of the following statements is *true?*
   a. The permanent mandibular second molars are erupted.
   b. There is no evidence of mandibular third molars.
   c. There are malpositioned maxillary canines.
   d. The primary maxillary first molars are still present.

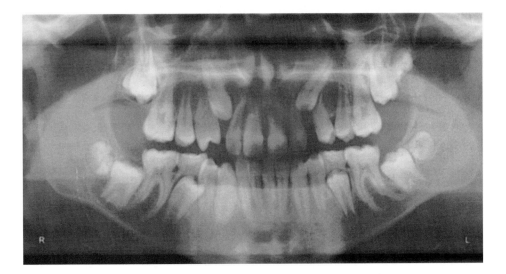

70. If you were mounting this film and the raised embossed dot was facing you, this film would be a _____ premolar view.
   a. maxillary right
   b. maxillary left
   c. mandibular right
   d. mandibular left

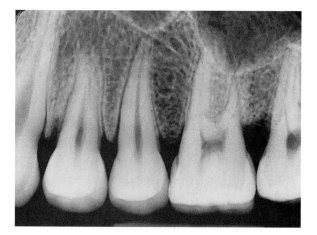

71. When mounting bitewing radiographs, mount them with the curve of Spee directed _____ toward the distal.
   a. upward
   b. downward

72. Most tooth roots curve toward the _____.
   a. mesial
   b. distal
   c. lingual
   d. buccal

73. If you were mounting this film and the raised embossed dot was facing you, this film would be
a _____ molar view.
   a. maxillary right
   b. maxillary left
   c. mandibular right
   d. mandibular left ✓

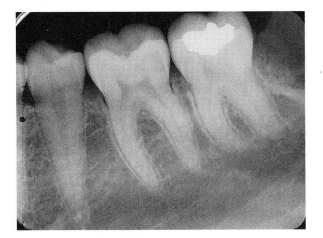

74. If you were mounting this film and the raised embossed dot was facing you, this film would be
a _____ molar view.
   a. maxillary right
   b. maxillary left ✓
   c. mandibular right
   d. mandibular left

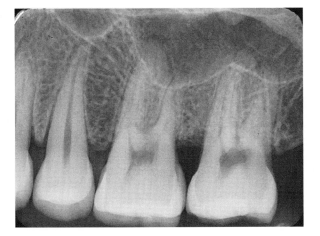

75. Incorrect vertical angulation can result in an image that is:
   a. elongated
   b. overlapped
   c. foreshortened
   d. both a and c

76. Because of the curvature of the arch, the optimal number of bitewings is _____.
   a. two
   b. four
   c. six
   d. eight

77. A two-film packet requires _____ exposure time as a one-film packet.
   a. the same
   b. half the time
   c, twice the time
   d. triple the time

78. The identification dot is used to:
   a. determine film orientation
   b. identify whether or not a film has been exposed
   c. identify the film speed
   d. identify the side of the film with an emulsion

79. In a film packet, the thin lead foil sheet is positioned _____.
   a. in front of the film
   b. behind the film
   c. in front of the paper film wrapper
   d. behind the paper film wrapper

80. Which of the following is a beam alignment device?
   a. Snap-A-Ray
   b. Stabe Bite Block
   c. EEZEE Grip
   d. precision film holder

81. The _____ allows for the positioning of the tubehead.
   a. control device
   b. exposure button
   c. extension arm
   d. exposure light

82. The acronym for the permitted lifetime accumulated dose is _____.
   a. MPD, maximum permissible dose
   b. MPD, maximum possible dose
   c. MAD, maximum accumulated dose
   d. MAD, maximum allowable dose

83. A _____ aids in stabilizing the film in the patient's mouth.
    a. PID
    b. control panel
    c. film holder
    d. cassette

84. To test the automatic film processor, _____ in the automatic processor.
    a. unwrap one film, expose it to light, and then process the film
    b. unwrap one film, do not expose it to light, and then process the film
    c. unwrap two unexposed films, expose one to light, and then process the exposed film
    d. unwrap two unexposed films, expose one to light, and then process both films

85. Which of the following may *not* be a radiographer?
    a. dentist
    b. dental assistant
    c. dental hygienist
    d. dental laboratory technician

86. The time interval between radiographic examinations for children should be:
    a. every 6 months
    b. every 12 months
    c. biannually
    d. based on the individual needs of the child

87. A patient with periodontal disease will likely require _____ radiographic examinations than a patient with a healthy periodontium.
    a. less frequent
    b. more frequent

88. Prior to radiation exposure for a minor, informed consent:
    a. must be obtained from an adult
    b. must be obtained from a legal guardian
    c. must be obtained from the patient
    d. may be waived if they have insurance

89. To avoid occupation exposure to radiation, which is the most critical for a dental radiographer?
    a. maintain an adequate distance
    b. have proper positioning of the patient
    c. use proper shielding
    d. avoid exposure to the primary beam

90. The _____ radiation received and the ____ the dose rate, the shorter is the latent period.
    a. less, slower
    b. less, faster
    c. more, slower
    d. more, faster

91. Which of the following changes will increase x-ray beam intensity?
   a. decreasing the kilovoltage peak
   b. decreasing the milliamperage
   c. decreasing the exposure time
   d. decreasing the source-to-film distance

92. The quantity of x-rays produced is controlled by _____.
   a. voltage
   b. kilovoltage
   c. kilovoltage peak
   d. milliamperage

93. What is the error in this film?
   a. reticulation
   b. fixer spots
   c. overlapped films
   d. fingerprints

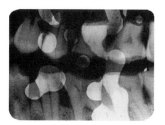

94. What is the error in this film?
   a. scratch mark
   b. reticulation
   c. roller marks
   d. fingerprints

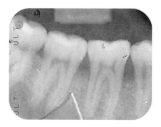

95. What is the error in this film?
  a. scratch mark
  b. elongation
  c. foreshortening
  d. fingerprints

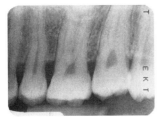

96. What is the manual processing error in this film?
  a. scratch mark
  b. reticulation
  c. developer cut off
  d. fixer cut off

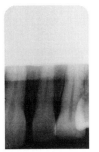

97. If the dot is facing the operator, this film shows the _____ region.
  a. mandibular right premolar
  b. mandibular right molar
  c. mandibular left premolar
  d. mandibular left molar

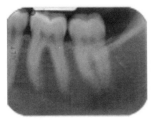

98. This film is an example of a _____ radiograph.
- **a.** periapical
- **b.** bitewing
- **c.** occlusal
- **d.** panoramic

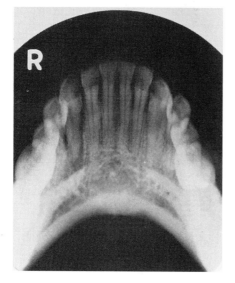

Review the figure below to answer questions 99 and 100.

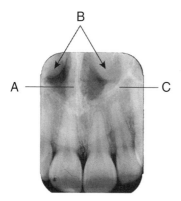

99. Which of the marked areas is the nasal septum?

100. Which of the marked areas is the floor of the nasal cavity?

Infection Control

Directions: Select the response that best answers each of the following questions. Only one response is correct.

1. If you opt not to receive a hepatitis B vaccination, you will be required to sign a(n):
   a. waiver that you will not ever request the vaccine
   b. waiver that if you change your mind you will assume the cost of the vaccine
   c. informed refusal that is kept on file in the dental office
   d. informed refusal that is sent to OSHA

2. All dental professionals must use surgical masks and protective eyewear to protect the eyes and face:
   a. only during surgical procedures
   b. only when treating patients of potential risk
   c. whenever spatter and aerosolized sprays of blood and saliva are likely
   d. as an option

3. All dental assistants involved in the direct provision of patient care must undergo routine training in:
   a. infection control, safety issues, and hazard communication
   b. charting, taking patients' vital signs, and using the office intercom system
   c. infection control, uniform sizing, and ordering of disposables
   d. hazardous waste management, charting, and application of dental dam

4. _____ occurs from a person previously contracting a disease and then recovering.
   a. Naturally acquired immunity
   b. Active natural immunity
   c. Artificially acquired immunity
   d. Inherited immunity

5. _____ immunity occurs when a vaccination is administered and the body forms antibodies in response to the vaccine.
   a. Active natural
   b. Active artificial
   c. Passive natural
   d. Passive artificial

6. A latent infection is best exemplified by which of the following?
   a. hepatitis D virus
   b. cold sore
   c. common cold
   d. pneumonia

7. Which of the following exemplifies an acute infection?
   a. hepatitis C virus
   b. cold sore
   c. common cold
   d. pneumonia

8. Microorganisms that produce disease in humans are known as:
   a. nonpathogenic
   b. pathogens
   c. pasteurized
   d. germs

9. A(n) _____ is a person who is unable to resist infection by a pathogen.
   a. infectious person
   b. susceptible host
   c. potential risk
   d. person of concern

10. An infection that occurs when the body's ability to resist diseases is weakened is a(n):
    a. chronic infection
    b. latent infection
    c. acute infection
    d. opportunistic infection

11. A disease that can be transmitted in some way from one host to another is a(n):
    a. infectious disease
    b. communicable disease
    c. contagious disease
    d. all of the above

12. The transmission of a disease through the skin, as with cuts or punctures, is _____ transmission.
    a. airborne
    b. parenteral
    c. indirect
    d. spatter

13. Which of the following would be considered the best method for determining whether there is proper sterilization function by a sterilizer?
    a. chemically treated tape used on packages that changes color
    b. viewing the temperature and pressure gauges
    c. biological spore test through a monitoring system

14. When the assistant prepares a package of hazardous infectious waste for disposal, which of the following statements is true?
    a. All infectious waste destined for disposal should be placed in closable, leak-proof containers or bags that are color-coded or labeled appropriately.
    b. Infectious waste should be burned in a local incinerator.
    c. Only the clinical assistant should manage the removal of infectious waste.

15. Protective eyewear should have _____.
    a. extra-thick lenses
    b. tinted lenses
    c. side shields
    d. spring-loaded ear rests

16. Exam gloves used during dental treatment can be made of:
    a. latex
    b. vinyl
    c. clear plastic
    d. both a and b

17. Infectious or regulated waste (biohazard) include all of the following *except* _____.
    a. blood and blood-soaked materials
    b. pathologic waste
    c. sharps
    d. x-ray wrappers

18. Which of the following statements is *not* true as they apply to the use of overgloves?
    a. Overgloves must be worn carefully to avoid contamination during handling with contamination procedure gloves.
    b. Overgloves are placed before the secondary procedure is performed and are removed before patient treatment is resumed.
    c. Overgloves are discarded after a single use.
    d. Overgloves are acceptable alone as a hand barrier in nonsurgical procedures.

19. During which of the following procedures would you use sterile surgical gloves?
    a. placement of a composite
    b. removal of a suture
    c. all bonding procedures
    d. mandibular resection

20. Which of the following statements is *not* an appropriate action for postexposure medical evaluation and follow-up?
    a. The employer must send the employee for medical evaluation, for which the employee must assume the cost.
    b. Give a copy of the OSHA standard to the health care professional.
    c. File an incident report.
    d. Assure that test results of source individual are given to the health care professional and that the health care professional informs the employee of these results confidentially.

21. Which of the following is a cause of sterilization failure?
    a. adequate space between packages in the autoclave
    b. using cloth wrappers in steam sterilizer
    c. using closed containers in steam or chemical vapor sterilizer
    d. using distilled water in a steam sterilizer

22. To prevent contamination of surfaces, which of the following techniques should be used?
    a. Place utility gloves prior to placement of appropriate surface covers.
    b. Apply appropriate surface covers before the surfaces have a chance to become contaminated with patient material.
    c. Place each cover surface directly under the cassette so the entire surface is not cluttered with protective covers.
    d. Always clean the underlying protected surface with a disinfectant.

23. An emergency action plan may be communicated orally if the workplace has fewer than _____ employees.
    a. 3
    b. 5
    c. 7
    d. 10

24. What is the maximum volume that a single container of alcohol-based hand rub solution placed within a dental treatment room can legally have?
    a. 250 ml
    b. 400 ml
    c. 2.0 L
    d. 5.0 L

25. All of the following surfaces *except* one may need to be cleaned and disinfected before each patient appointment. Which one is the exception?
    a. drawer pulls and top edges of drawers that may be used
    b. floors
    c. high-volume evacuation connector
    d. handpiece connectors

26. A tip for protecting dental instruments includes all of the following *except* _____.
    a. clean as soon as possible after use
    b. rinse well after cleaning
    c. use distilled or deionized water in steam sterilizers
    d. dry items before processing through steam under pressure sterilizers

27. Protective eyewear should have:
    a. extra thick lenses
    b. tinted lenses
    c. magnification provisions
    d. side shields

28. The costs associated with hepatitis B vaccines of at risk employees are:
    a. the responsibility of the employees themselves
    b. to be paid by the employer
    c. usually covered by a grant from OSHA
    d. paid for by the employee's health insurance policy

29. Bacteria that make acids are called _____.
    a. aerobic
    b. nonaerobic
    c. acidogenic
    d. viral

30. Bacteria that die in the presence of oxygen are known as _____.
    a. aerobic
    b. nonaerobic
    c. acidogenic
    d. fimbriae

31. When an assistant transfers a microbe from one patient to his or her hand and then to another patient's mouth, this transmission is referred to as _____.
    a. direct contact
    b. indirect contact
    c. airborne transmission
    d. droplet transmission

32. A(n) _____ is a protein manufactured in the body that binds to and destroys microbes and other antigens.
    a. antibiotic
    b. antibody
    c. microbe
    d. allergen

33. The strength of an organism in its ability to produce disease is:
    a. virulence
    b. bioburden
    c. pathogens
    d. infectious disease

34. Another name for airborne transmission is:
    a. aerosol
    b. mist
    c. droplet infection
    d. all of the above

35. Pathogens that are carried in the blood and body fluids of infected individuals and that can be transmitted to others are referred to as:
    a. bloodborne
    b. parenteral
    c. virulent
    d. acquired

36. Recommendations concerning gloves would fall under which of the following categories of infection control practices that directly relate to dental radiography procedures?
    a. surface disinfection
    b. protective attire and barrier techniques
    c. sterilization or disinfection of instruments
    d. maintenance of the environment

37. Protective clothing:
    a. must prevent skin exposure when contact with blood or other bodily fluids is anticipated
    b. must prevent mucous membrane exposure when contact with blood or other bodily fluids is anticipated
    c. should be worn home and laundered daily
    d. both a and b

38. Which of the following is an infectious disease?
    a. malfunctioning of the pancreas
    b. abnormal growth of body cells
    c. tissue damage caused by a microorganism
    d. an allergic reaction to a substance

39. The substance in a vaccine that stimulates an immune response is called an _____.
  a. antibody
  b. antibiotic
  c. antigen
  d. acidogen

40. How does HIV cause AIDS?
  a. it destroys the liver
  b. it diminishes the ability to control muscles
  c. it paralyzes the organs
  d. it destroys the body's defenses against diseases

41. The risk of getting HIV as a dental assistant is:
  a. very high
  b. high
  c. moderate
  d. low

42. When using medical latex or vinyl gloves, _____.
  a. gloves may be rewashed between patients and reused until damaged
  b. nonsterile gloves are recommended for examinations and nonsurgical procedures
  c. hands should not be washed before gloving
  d. hands should not be washed between patients

43. _____ is defined as the absence of pathogens, or disease-causing microorganisms.
  a. Antiseptic
  b. Antibiotic
  c. Antiinfective
  d. Asepsis

44. Antiseptic is:
  a. the absence of pathogens, or disease-causing microorganisms
  b. a substance that inhibits the growth of bacteria
  c. the use of a chemical or physical procedure to inhibit or destroy pathogens
  d. the act of sterilizing

45. A disease arising from within the body that is caused by opportunistic microorganisms already present in the body is referred to as a(n) _____ infection.
  a. nosocomial
  b. exogenous
  c. endogenous
  d. opportunistic

46. Which of the following agents is *not* tuberculocidal?
  a. iodophor
  b. quaternary ammonium compound
  c. phenolic
  d. glutaraldehyde·

47. When can a liquid sterilant/high-level disinfectant achieve sterilization?
    a. only when the solution is used at temperatures above 121° C
    b. when the solution is used only for longer exposure times
    c. as soon as the minimal exposure time is reached
    d. only when the solution is used under pressure

48. Which of the following may be used for surface disinfectant in the dental office?
    a. iodophors
    b. ethyl alcohol
    c. isopropyl alcohol
    d. iodine

49. Sterilizers such as autoclaves are preset to reach a maximum steam temperature of ____ degrees Fahrenheit and a pressure of ____ pounds per square inch (psi).
    a. 500, 40
    b. 350, 10 to 25
    c. 250, 15 to 30
    d. 400, 25

50. When using the _____ method of sterilization, instruments must be absolutely dry or they will rust.
    a. chemical vapor
    b. cold sterile
    c. steam autoclave
    d. flash sterilization

51. Which of the following is considered to be a semicritical instrument in radiography?
    a. the exposure button
    b. the x-ray control panel
    c. the lead apron
    d. x-ray film holding device

52. The stage of an infectious disease when the patient's symptoms begin to subside is called _____.
    a. acute
    b. prodromal
    c. incubation
    d. convalescent

53. This method of sterilization requires good ventilation.
    a. steam under pressure
    b. cold chemical/immersion disinfection
    c. unsaturated chemical vapor
    d. flash sterilization

54. Which of the following microbes are well known for causing periodic recurrences after the initial infection?
    a. influenza viruses
    b. rubella viruses
    c. human herpes viruses
    d. gonorrhea

55. Which government agency requires employers to protect their employees from exposure to blood and saliva at work?
   a. FDA
   b. EPA
   c. CDC ✓
   d. OSHA ✓

56. If a thorough job of cleaning or sterilizing reusable hand instruments is *not* accomplished, this will contribute to which pathway of cross–contamination in the office?
   a. patient to dental team
   b. patient to patient
   c. dental team to patient
   d. community to office

57. When using this method of sterilization, the exposure time varies as to whether the instruments are wrapped or unwrapped.
   a. steam under pressure
   b. cold chemical/immersion disinfection
   c. unsaturated chemical vapor
   d. flash sterilization

58. From the list below, select the best procedure for caring for orthodontic wire.
   a. steam under pressure with emulsion
   b. steam under pressure without emulsion
   c. sharps container
   d. spray/wipe/spray with surface disinfectant

59. From the list below, select the best procedure for caring for a pair of crown and collar scissors.
   a. steam under pressure with emulsion
   b. steam under pressure without emulsion
   c. cold chemical/immersion
   d. spray/wipe/spray with surface disinfectant

60. From the list below, select the best procedure for caring for a pair of surgical suction tips.
   a. steam under pressure with emulsion
   b. steam under pressure without emulsion
   c. cold chemical/immersion
   d. spray/wipe/spray with surface disinfectant

61. Which of the following is the recommended scheme for immunization against hepatitis B?
   a. injections at 0, 1, and 6 months
   b. an injection now and then another one in 1 month
   c. injections at 0, 1, and 3 months
   d. an injection now and another one 6 months later

62. From the list below, select the best procedure for caring for a mandrel.
   a. steam under pressure with emulsion
   b. steam under pressure without emulsion
   c. cold chemical/immersion
   d. discard

63. The intent of handwashing is to remove:
    a. transient flora
    b. normal flora
    c. transient and normal flora

64. From the list below, select the best procedure for caring for a pair of protective glasses.
    a. steam under pressure with emulsion
    b. steam under pressure without emulsion
    c. cold chemical/immersion
    d. spray/wipe/spray with surface disinfectant

65. What is the active agent in hand rubs acceptable for use in dental offices?
    a. triclosan
    b. chlorhexidine
    c. iodophor
    d. alcohol

66. Which type of sterilization used in the dental office requires the longest processing time?
    a. steam autoclave
    b. chemical vapor
    c. dry heat sterilization
    d. chemical liquid sterilization

67. Immersion in a chemical liquid sterilant requires at least ____ hour(s) of contact time for sterilization to occur.
    a. 1
    b. 10
    c. 5
    d. 24

68. Instruments have been in a liquid sterilant for 2 hours. The assistant adds another batch of instruments. Which of the following statements addresses this situation?
    a. Two completion times will be used: one for the first set of instrument and the other for the second batch.
    b. The total time will be 24 hours for the entire batch.
    c. The total time will be 1 hour for the entire batch.
    d. Retiming must begin again once the second batch has been added to the original instruments.

69. The ideal instrument processing area should be:
    a. large enough for several assistants to work at one time
    b. dedicated only to instrument processing
    c. part of the treatment rooms and dental laboratory
    d. outside the dental suite

70. What should the work flow pattern be for processing contaminated instruments?
    a. dirty, to sterile, to storage
    b. dirty, to clean, to sterile, to storage
    c. dirty, to preclean, to clean, to storage
    d. dirty, to preclean, to clean, to sterilize, to storage

71. Which of the following methods of precleaning dental instruments should be avoided?
 a. instrument washing machines
 b. rinsing in a holding solution
 c. hand scrubbing
 d. ultrasonic cleaning

72. Which statement is *not* true about an ultrasonic cleaner?
 a. It aids in precleaning.
 b. It prevents injuries to staff members.
 c. It disinfects and sterilizes.
 d. It is efficient.

73. After instruments have completed the cleaning cycle of the ultrasonic cleaner, they should be:
 a. wiped and dried
 b. rinsed with clear water
 c. placed in the sterilizer
 d. stored

74. The last of the PPEs to be put on before patient treatment begins is(are):
 a. gown
 b. mask
 c. gloves
 d. eyeglasses

75. Heavy utility gloves should be used:
 a. for all intraoral procedures
 b. for radiographic processing
 c. for entering data on the computer
 d. to work with contaminated instruments

76. Which of the following statements is *not* true as it relates to the use of glutaraldehyde as an immersion disinfectant/sterilant?
 a. It may be used as a high-level disinfectant or a sterilant by following the manufacturer's guidelines for immersion time.
 b. It is not toxic and may be used in a closed environment.
 c. It should not be used as a surface disinfectant.
 d. Always keep the container lid closed.

77. The sterilization process is best described as being:
 a. bactericidal
 b. sporicidal
 c. tuberculocidal
 d. virucidal

78. The process that kills disease-causing microorganisms, but not necessarily all microbial life, is defined as:
 a. precleaning
 b. sterilization
 c. disinfection
 d. cleaning

79. The best way to determine that sterilization has actually occurred is to use:
    a. process integrators
    b. biologic monitors
    c. process indicators
    d. color-changing sterilization bags or tape

80. Low-level disinfection can be used for:
    a. clinical contact surfaces
    b. heat-sensitive reusable items
    c. housekeeping surfaces such as floors or walls
    d. dental unit

81. Patient care instruments are categorized into various classifications. Into which classification would instruments such as impression trays, dental mouth mirror, and amalgam condenser be placed?
    a. critical
    b. semicritical
    c. noncritical

82. Which of the following does *not* minimize the amount of dental aerosols and spatter generated during treatment?
    a. preprocedural mouth rinse
    b. saliva ejectors
    c. rubber dams
    d. high-volume evacuation

83. Which of the following microbes are *not* killed by intermediate-level disinfection?
    a. bacterial spores
    b. tuberculosis agent
    c. both a and b
    d. neither a nor b

84. Which of the following is *not* a recommended PPE for cleaning and disinfecting a dental treatment room?
    a. mask
    b. utility gloves
    c. latex gloves
    d. protective eyewear

85. OSHA requires a *minimum* of training of dental personnel in all of the following areas *except* _____.
    a. the Bloodborne Pathogens Standard
    b. the Hazard Communication Standard
    c. specialty safety standards
    d. general safety standards

86. Which of the following statements is *true* as it relates to the environmental infection control in a clinical area?
    a. Change barriers twice daily.
    b. Avoid the use of carpet and cloth-upholstered furnishings.
    c. Use isopropyl alcohol on fixed surfaces.
    d. Avoid barriers on the dental unit.

87. The Organization for Safety and Asepsis Procedures identifies the classification of clinical touch surfaces to include which of the following?
    a. instrument trays, handpiece holders, and countertops
    b. light handles, dental unit controls, and chair switches
    c. unit master switch, fixed cabinetry, and patient record
    d. telephone, assistant stool, and fixed cabinetry

88. Chemicals that destroy or inactivate most species of pathogenic microorganisms on inanimate surfaces are called:
    a. disinfectants
    b. sterilants
    c. antiseptics
    d. antigermicidal

89. Who determines the hazards of a chemical?
    a. employer
    b. employees
    c. manufacturer
    d. distributor

90. When a denture is being sent to a commercial laboratory, it should be _____.
    a. disinfected before being sent out
    b. packaged and sent to the laboratory for later disinfection
    c. disinfected after being received back from the laboratory
    d. disinfected before being sent out and after being received back from the laboratory

91. A victim who feels the effects of a chemical spill immediately, with symptoms of dizziness, headache, nausea, and vomiting, is experiencing:
    a. chronic chemical toxicity
    b. acute chemical toxicity
    c. chemical resistance
    d. mild exposure

92. _____ is considered regulated waste and requires special disposal.
    a. Human tissue
    b. Food
    c. Saliva-soaked gauze
    d. Used anesthetic carpule

93. The office safety supervisor should check the contents of the emergency kit to determine that the contents are in place and within the expiration date _____.
    a. weekly
    b. monthly
    c. biannually
    d. annually

94. Which of the following statements is *true* concerning cleaning and disinfection of the dental unit and environmental surfaces?
   a. An intermediate-level disinfectant is recommended.
   b. A low-level disinfectant is recommended.
   c. EPA-registered chemical germicides labeled as both hospital disinfectants and tuberculocidals are classified as low-level disinfectants.
   d. Both a and c are true.

95. All waste containers that hold potentially infectious materials must:
   a. have a red bag
   b. be labeled with the biohazard symbol
   c. have special disposal
   d. be labeled as infectious waste

96. The OSHA Hazard Communications Standard requires employers to do all *except* _____.
   a. tell employees about the identity and hazards of chemicals in the workplace
   b. implement a hazard communication program
   c. maintain accurate and thorough MSDS records
   d. submit annual hair sample results of all employees

97. A DHCW transfers a small amount of cavity medication into a smaller container for use on a patient at chairside. A new label must be placed on that container if:
   a. more material is required during the course of treating that patient
   b. the chemical material is not used up at the conclusion of an 8-hour work shift
   c. the patient recently tested positive for HIV
   d. no MSDS can be found on file for that material

98. When recapping the needle, the dental assistant should use any of the following methods *except* _____.
   a. a one-handed scoop method
   b. a mechanical device specifically designed to hold the needle for recapping
   c. any safety feature that is fixed, provides a barrier between the assistant's hands and the needle following use, and allows the assistant's hands to remain behind the needle
   d. a two-handed scoop method for maximum control

99. During which phase is it likely the microbes begin to multiply and form a spreading film or layer on the tubing walls of dental unit hosing?
   a. initial
   b. accumulation
   c. release

100. The ADA, OSAP, and CDC recommend that the dental assistant:
   a. flush the dental unit waterlines for 30 seconds each morning and again at the end of the day
   b. flush the dental unit waterlines for 20 to 30 seconds each morning and between patients
   c. flush the dental unit waterlines 60 seconds each morning and 30 seconds after treating an HIV-infected patient
   d. flush the dental unit waterlines for 30 seconds each hour of the day

Answer Keys and Rationales

TEST 2

General Chairside

1. A patient displaying hypertension would have a blood pressure of about:
   d. Normal blood pressure for an adult is less than 120/80 mm Hg. Hypertension is considered to be 140/90 mm Hg and above.

2. A patient presents appearing "flushed" and states that he has an infection. Which temperature would most likely be measured?
   d. A normal temperature is 98.6° F. If a patient presented with the symptoms as listed, the temperature would likely be higher than 99.6° F, and thus the best answer is 102° F.

3. The normal blood pressure classification for adults is:
   a. Normal blood pressure for an adult is less than 120/80 mm Hg.

4. The most common site for taking a patient's pulse when performing cardiopulmonary resuscitation is the:
   b. The carotid artery is the most common site for taking a patient's pulse when administering CPR. This pulse is found by placing two fingers alongside the patient's larynx on the side of the neck nearest you. This makes it a quick procedure during CPR.

5. Consent is:
   b. Consent is a voluntary acceptance or agreement to what is planned or done by another person. Consent is given freely by the patient.

6. Using Black's classification of cavities, a pit lesion on the buccal surface of molars and premolars is considered a Class _____ restoration or cavity.
   a. A Class I restoration or cavity is described as a pit lesion on the buccal surface of molars and premolars using Black's classification of cavities.

7. The abbreviation used in the progress notes or chart to indicate a mesioocclusodistal lesion would be:
   c. Each surface is given an initial, and in the naming of this restoration, the surfaces are in the sequence of mesial, occlusal, and distal—thus MOD.

8. The tooth-numbering system that gives each of the four quadrants its own tooth bracket made up of a vertical and horizontal line is referred to as the:
   b. In the Palmer Notation System, each of the four quadrants is given its own tooth bracket made up of a vertical and a horizontal line. The Palmer method is a shorthand diagram of the teeth as if viewing the patient's teeth from the outside. The teeth in the right quadrant would have the vertical midline bracket to the right of the tooth numbers or letters, just as when looking at the patient. The midline is to the right of the teeth in the right quadrant. The number or letter assigned to each tooth depends on the position relative to the midline. Central incisors, closest to the midline, have the smallest number (1) for permanent teeth and the letter A for primary teeth. The teeth are then numbered to the distal, 1 through 8 for permanent teeth and A through E for primary teeth.

9. Any tooth that remains unerupted in the jaw beyond the time at which it should normally erupt is referred to as being:
   b. An impacted tooth is one that is so positioned in the jawbone that eruption is not possible.

10. A tray is set up from _____ to _____.
    a. A tray is set up from left to right based on how instruments are transferred and used throughout a dental procedure.

11. The "A" in the ABCDs of basic life support stands for:
    c. In all emergency situations the rescuers must promptly initiate the ABCDs of basic life support: *airway, breathing, circulation,* and *defibrillation.*

12. An arrow used as a charting symbol indicates which of the following?
    b. An arrow indicates the tooth has drifted either distally or mesially.

13. A periodontal probe is an example of which type of instrument?
    a. A periodontal probe is an examination instrument used to measure the depth of the gingival sulcus.

14. A patient, aged 78, presents for a partial denture examination. She appears to weigh about 100 lb, is frail, has a rather slow gait, and indicates she has no health contraindications, is only taking some vitamins, but does have some slight hearing problems. When her blood pressure is taken, it is likely to be:
    a. A blood pressure reading of 106/52 mm Hg is indicative of a person the age of this patient with no health history contraindications.

15. The normal pulse rate for a resting adult is:
    c. The normal pulse rate for an adult is between 60 and 100 beats per minute. It is more rapid for a child.

16. A new patient tells you that her blood pressure normally is low. If this is true, her blood pressure could be which of the following?
    a. Normal blood pressure for an adult is 102/80 mm Hg or slightly lower. Hypotension would be a lower reading.

17. A patient displaying hypertension would have a blood pressure of about:
    d. Hypertension is indicated at stage 1 as 140 to 159 mm Hg for the systolic reading and 90 to 99 mm Hg for the diastolic reading. Stage 2 is 160+ mm Hg for the systolic reading and 100+ mm Hg for the diastolic reading.

18. A patient with hypothermia would have a temperature of:
    a. Hypothermia is body temperature that is below normal, generally between 78° and 90° F.

19. The automated external defibrillator (AED) is used for all *except* to _____.
    b. The AED is basically an advanced computer microprocessor that assesses the patient's cardiac rhythm and identifies any rhythm for which a shock is indicated. The shock is a massive jolt of electricity that is sent to the heart muscle to reestablish the proper rhythm of the heart.

20. _____ can be life threatening and is indicated by nausea and vomiting, shortness of breath, and loss of consciousness.
    a. Anaphylaxis is one form of a type I allergic or hypersensitivity reaction to an allergenic antigen. This condition can be life threatening and is indicated by nausea and vomiting, shortness of breath, and/or loss of consciousness.

21. The respirations of a patient who is hyperventilating will be exemplified by:
    c. A patient who is hyperventilating will display excessively long, rapid breaths. This is a frequent finding in patients with asthma, metabolic acidosis, or pulmonary embolism and also in anxiety-induced states.

22. The respiration pattern of a patient in a state of tachypnea has:
    b. A patient with nervous tachypnea will display a respiratory rate of 40 or more per minute and the breaths will be excessively short and rapid.

23. The symbol on tooth No. 31 indicates it is:
    b. The symbol on tooth No. 31 indicates that it has drifted distally.

24. The symbol on tooth No. 8 indicates it will need to have:
    b. There is a periapical abscess on this tooth with the mesioincisal angle fractured. The patient will need to have endodontic treatment and then a restoration to replace the mesioincisal angle.

25. The symbol between teeth No. 24 and No. 25 indicates:
    d. The two vertical lines indicate the presence of a diastema or a space that is wider than normal between two teeth.

26. The symbol on tooth No. 23 indicates that this tooth:
    b. An implant is indicated commonly by drawing horizontal lines through the root or roots of the tooth or teeth.

27. The symbol on tooth No. 3 indicates that this tooth:
    a. A common symbol, S, is used to indicate the presence of a sealant.

28. How many permanent teeth have erupted?
    b. On this chart, 10 permanent teeth have erupted: all of the permanent central incisors, the mandibular lateral incisors, and all four permanent first molars.

29. How many permanent teeth are present on the mandible?
    a. All four permanent incisors are present as well as the two permanent first molars.

30. The examination technique in which the examiner uses his or her fingers and hands to feel for size, texture, and consistency of hard and soft tissue is called:
    b. Palpation is the examination technique in which the examiner uses the fingers and hands to feel for size, texture, and consistency of hard and soft tissue. Detection is the act or process of discovering tooth imperfections or decay, while probing is using a slender, flexible instrument to explore and measure the periodontal pocket. The extraoral exam is a visual inspection of the landmarks outside the oral cavity.

31. Which of the following statements is *not* true as it relates to a patient's respiration?
    d. This statement is not true. It is in reverse. Normally respiration counts are lower per minute than a pulse rate.

32. Most local anesthetic agents used for dental procedures are:
    b. Intermediate-acting local anesthetic agents last 120 to 240 minutes. Most local anesthetic agents are in this group and are used for dental procedures.

33. In the United States, nitrous oxide gas lines are color-coded _____ and oxygen lines are color-coded _____.
    d. In the United States, nitrous oxide gas lines are color-coded blue and oxygen gas lines are color-coded green. Other countries may have different color codes.

34. The dental assistant's responsibility in an emergency situation is to:
    d. The dental assistant works with the rest of the dental team to recognize the symptoms and signs of a significant medical complaint and to provide appropriate support in implementing emergency procedures. The dental assistant does not diagnose a condition in the emergency situation.

35. A condition called _____ will result if an alginate impression absorbs additional water by being stored in water or in a very wet paper towel.
    c. The condition in which an alginate impression absorbs additional water is inbibition. Syneresis would result in the impression shrinking and becoming distorted. Alginate is a type of hydrocolloid impression material. Polymerization is the curing reaction of elastomeric impression materials.

36. A patient who displays symptoms of intermittent blinking, mouth movements, blank stare, and nonresponsiveness to surroundings may be displaying symptoms of:
    a. Common symptoms of a petit mal seizure are intermittent blinking, mouth movements, blank stare, and being not responsive to surroundings. This condition does not result in loss of consciousness, as does the grand mal seizure.

37. The water-to-powder ratio generally used for an adult mandibular impression is ____ measures of water, _____ scoops of powder.
    d. The water-to-powder ratio used for an adult mandibular impression is generally two measures of water and two scoops of powder.

38. The RDAs are the levels of essential nutrients that are needed by individuals on a daily basis. RDA stands for:
    a. The Food and Nutrition Board of the National Academy of Sciences have determined the RDA levels of essential nutrients that are needed by individuals on a daily basis. These are referred to as the recommended dietary allowances.

39. The only nutrients that can build and repair body tissues are:
    a. The primary function of proteins is to build and repair body tissues.

40. _____ can prevent cholesterol from oxidizing and damaging arteries.
    d. In addition to lowering the dietary intake of cholesterol, increasing the intake of antioxidants may be beneficial. Antioxidant vitamins are A and E and beta-carotene. Many fruits and vegetables also contain naturally occurring antioxidants.

41. The retromolar area is reproduced in the ____ ____ impression.
    b. The retromolar area, comprised of the lingual frenum, tongue space, and mylohyoid ridge, is reproduced in the mandibular impression. The hard palate and tuberosities are reproduced in the maxillary impression.

42. Which of the following instruments would be used to measure the depth of the gingival sulcus?
    a. A periodontal probe is an instrument with marked calibrations on the working tip that allows for measuring the depth of the gingival sulcus.

43. Which of the following instruments has sharp, round, angular tips used to detect tooth anomalies?
    b. The cowhorn explorer is the only one of these instruments with rounded tips. Its sharp tip enables the operator to detect anomalies in the tooth.

44. Which instrument is commonly used to scale surfaces in the anterior region of the mouth?
    c. The straight sickle scaler can only be used in the anterior region of the mouth because of its design. To scale the posterior teeth with a sickle scaler, the modified version would need to be used.

45. Which instrument is used to scale deep periodontal pockets or furcation areas?
    b. The Gracey scaler is designed with multiple bends in the shank and a fine cutting edge to enable the tip to be placed into deep periodontal pockets and furcation areas.

46. In the drawing below, which area stabilizes the clamp to the tooth.
    d. The four prongs in d. grasp the tooth, providing stability to the clamp once it is in place.

47. When the operator is working in the labial of tooth No. 9, the HVE tip is held:
    b. By placing the HVE tip on the lingual of this tooth, the assistant will be able to efficiently remove fluids and not interfere with the operator's handpiece.

48. A right-handed dentist is doing a preparation on 30MO. The dental assistant places the HVE tip:
    c. The HVE tip is placed on the surface of the tooth nearest the assistant, thus the tip would be placed on the lingual of No. 30.

49. The angle of the bevel of the HVE tip should always be:
    a. By placing the tip parallel to the buccal or lingual surface of the tooth, the assistant is able to remove fluids from the mouth more efficiently.

50. Which of the following is a thermoplastic material used to stabilize an anterior clamp?
    c. Dental compound is a rigid thermoplastic impression material that can be used on a clamp to stabilize it.

51. The wooden wedge is placed in the gingival embrasure area for Class II restorations to accomplish all *except* which of the following?
    a. The matrix band is used to provide a missing proximal wall, and the wedge then adapts the band to the cervical margin in order to prevent overhangs and maintain proximal contact.

52. Which of the following techniques could be used for caries removal?
    c. The instruments of choice would be the No. 2 RA and spoon excavator. Slower speed or manual removal is more efficient when removing soft carious material from the tooth.

53. Select the instrument that will be used to carve the distal surface of an amalgam restoration placed on 30DO.
    d. An instrument such as the Hollenback or Ward's carver is used to adequately carve the distal or smooth surface.

54. From the photograph below, select the instrument that would be used to attach to the rubber dam clamps.
    d. Instrument d is a rubber dam clamp forceps, and it is used to attach to a rubber dam clamp for easy placement of the clamp onto the tooth.

55. Which of the following instruments is a Hedstrom file?
    c. A Hedstrom file is shaped like a cone with a pointed tip and triangular edges.

56. Which of the photographs below illustrates an orthodontic hemostat?
    a. This orthodontic hemostat is used to hold and place materials such as separators and ligatures. They have gripping and locking capabilities.

57. Which instrument would be used to check for an overhang on a newly placed restoration?
    d. An explorer is the instrument of choice to determine the presence of an overhang. Its sharp tip will enable the operator to detect any anomaly in the restoration.

58. Which of the following instruments would be the least likely to be used for placing a cavity liner?
    d. The first three instruments are finer and easier to use to place a cavity liner. The condenser is bulkier for something as delicate as a liner but could be used in placing a base.

59. Under which of the following conditions would the shade for an anterior esthetic restoration *not* be selected?
    b. The shade selection should be completed before cavity preparation as the tooth may dry out and not appear as natural in color as prior to the preparation and cavity medication.

60. At what time can the final polish of a light-cured composite be accomplished?
  d. When using a composite material as a restoration, it may be finished as soon as the material has polymerized. Special finishing disks and points are available for finishing the restoration immediately without any deleterious effect on the restoration.

61. Which of the following would *not* be used for smooth surface carving in an amalgam procedure?
  c. The cleoid discoid carver is designed for use on the occlusal surface, not smooth surfaces such as the buccal, lingual, mesial, and distal.

62. Which of the following endodontic instruments is used to curette the inside of the tooth to the base of the pulp chamber?
  a. The long shank on an endodontic spoon enables the operator to curette the inside of the tooth to the base of the pulp chamber most efficiently.

63. Using the operating zones based on the "clock concept," the assistant's zone for a right-handed operator is:
  a. For a right-handed operator, the assistant is seated in the 2 to 4 o'clock position. Unlike the doctor's position, the assistant's position remains the same regardless of the arch being treated.

64. A finger rest that stabilizes the hand so that there is less possibility of slipping or traumatizing the tissue in the mouth is known as a _____.
  c. A fulcrum is a finger rest used when holding an instrument or a handpiece for a specified time. It provides safe practice for the operator.

65. Which of the following types of anesthesia produce a state of unconsciousness?
  d. General anesthesia is a controlled state of unconsciousness characterized by loss of protective reflexes, including the ability to maintain an airway independently and to respond appropriately to physical stimulation.

66. A cotton roll remains attached to the buccal mucosa after treatment has been completed. The safest way to remove the cotton roll is to:
  b. By moistening the cotton roll with water from the a/w syringe, the cotton roll can be removed easily without any discomfort to the patient.

67. The time from when the local anesthetic takes complete effect until the complete reversal of anesthesia is the _____ of the anesthetic agent.
  a. The duration of an anesthetic is from the onset of its effectiveness until the effect is reversed.

68. The lengths of the needles used in dentistry for local anesthesia administration are:
  b. The common sizes for needles used in dentistry for anesthetic administration are the 1 inch and 1⅝ inch.

69. The stage of anesthesia when the patient passes through excitement and becomes calm, feels no pain or sensation, and soon becomes unconscious is referred to as stage ___ of anesthesia.
  c. Stage III is the stage of anesthesia that begins when the patient becomes calm after stage II. The patient feels no pain or sensation.

70. The most common type of attachment for fixed orthodontic appliances is the:
  b. The bonded bracket is accepted as the most common type of attachment for fixed appliances.

71. When a health contraindication is present that prevents the use of a vasoconstrictor, the retraction cord is impregnated with _____ and the cord may have a _____ agent applied to it to control bleeding.
  d. Aluminum chloride is used instead of epinephrine in retraction cord when a health contraindication is evident. It may have a hemostatic agent applied to it to control bleeding at the treatment site.

72. The procedural tray shown below is used to:
  b. This tray is used to fit and cement orthodontic bands. Instruments such as the band seater and band pusher are used specifically for this procedure.

73. The instruments shown below from left to right are:
    c. The bird beak pliers, contouring pliers, and Weingart utility pliers are common to orthodontic procedures.

74. A nonsurgical technique that uses a sterile flat-ended brush to gather the surface cells from a suspect oral lesion is a(n) _____ biopsy.
    c. An exfoliative procedure is noninvasive and uses a sterile flat-ended brush to gather the surface cells from a suspect oral lesion.

75. The scalpel blade that resembles a bird's beak is a:
    b. A No. 12 scalpel blade is a popular scalpel blade used in a variety of dental procedures. It is easily recognized by its bird beak shape.

76. The ideal candidate for dental implants meets which of the following criteria?
    d. To be a candidate for an implant, the site must be in good health and have adequate alveolar bone for support. In addition, the patient must be willing to commit to conscientious oral hygiene and regular dental visits.

77. Which tissues are those that surround the root of the tooth?
    a. Periradicular tissues are those tissues that surround the root of a tooth. Periapical refers to the apex only of the tooth, gingival refers to gingival only, and osseous to bone.

78. The process of removing bacteria, necrotic tissue, and organic debris from the root canal is called:
    c. To debride is to remove foreign material and dead or damaged tissue from a wound.

79. From the photograph below, which instrument is a K-type file?
    b. The K-type file has a twisted design and is used in the initial debridement of the canal and in the later stages of shaping and contouring the canal.

80. Which of the following is *not* a surgical procedure performed to remove defects or restore normal contours to the bone?
    d. The first three answers all refer to some form of surgery to be performed on the bone to either remove defects or restore normal contours to the bone. A gingivoplasty is the reshaping and recontouring of gingival tissues.

81. _____ is a small rubber, silicone, or plastic device that is slid onto an endodontic instrument to prevent perforation of the apex during instrumentation.
    c. A stop is placed on the file to indicate its working length. This will aid in preventing perforation of the apex during instrumentation.

82. A dentist with a license in the specialty of dentistry that is involved in the diagnosis and treatment of the supporting tissues of the teeth is a(n) _____.
    b. A periodontist is a specialist concerned with the treatment of diseases of the tissues surrounding the teeth.

83. A condition of periodontal disease when the gingival tissues migrate away from the tooth, leaving portions of the roots of the teeth exposed below the cementoenamel junction, is called _____.
    b. Gingival recession is a condition when the gingival tissues migrate away from the tooth, leaving clefts, or recession, on portions of the roots of the teeth. The exposed tissue extends below the cementoenamel junction.

84. Vertical bitewing radiographs are especially valuable in periodontics to determine the _____.
    d. A vertical bitewing is particularly valuable because it can accurately depict the bone height along the root surface, and the vertical bitewing is excellent for determining the extent of crestal bone loss.

85. Indications for use of an ultrasonic scaler include all of the following *except* _____:
    d. The use of an ultrasonic scaler is contraindicated with a patient who has a pacemaker.

86. Which of the following is *not* an advantage of laser surgery in periodontics?
    d. There are many advantages to the use of laser surgery in periodontics, and although there may be a reduction in swelling, scarring, and pain, pain is not eliminated.

87. A double-ended knife with kidney-shaped blades commonly used in periodontal surgery is known as a(n):
    b. The Kirkland knife is a common periodontal surgical instrument that is double ended with kidney-shaped blades.

88. In which of the following procedures could the patient be placed in an upright position?
    d. Although it is a procedure that could be done in a supine position, most operators prefer to take diagnostic impressions in an upright position to avoid any problems with the impression materials going into the throat area.

89. Select the straight elevator.
    b. The straight elevator is a single-ended surgical instrument as shown in b. The first instrument on the tray is a periosteal elevator.

90. Which instrument would be used to debride the interior of the tooth socket after an extraction?
    d. The surgical curette is used to debride the tooth socket following an extraction.

91. A patient is to take a medication three times a day. The prescription will indicate to the pharmacy that it is taken:
    b. The Latin, *ter in die (tid),* means "three times a day."

92. If the signature line on a prescription states *1 tab QID prn pain,* it indicates that the patient would take the medication:
    c. The Latin, *quater in die,* means "four times a day," and prn, *pro re nata,* "as circumstances may require or as necessary." Thus, the patient is directed to take one tablet four times a day as needed for pain.

93. An antibiotic _____.
    c. The primary function of an antibiotic is to kill or inhibit the growth of microorganisms.

94. An example of an anticoagulant is _____.
    d. According to the manufacturer's description, Coumadin is an anticoagulant, or blood thinner.

95. Which is the correct sequence for placing sealants?
    c. According to common manufacturer's directions, the process for placing a sealant is to clean, isolate, etch.

96. The type of implant used primarily on patients with severely resorbed ridges, and only if there is no other option is _____.
    a. The transosteal implant is inserted through the inferior border of the mandible and into the edentulous area. The implants are used primarily on patients with severely resorbed ridges, and only if there are no other options. An endosteal implant is surgically placed into the bone and used to support, stabilize, and retain removable dentures, fixed bridges, and single-tooth implants. A subperiosteal implant is used to support a mandibular complete denture, primarily for patients who do not have sufficient alveolar ridge to support an endosteal implant.

97. Addition of very warm water to an alginate mix will cause the setting time to be:
    b. When warm water is added to an alginate mix, the material will set faster; thus, the setting time is decreased.

98. A negative reproduction of the patient's dental arch is referred to as a(n):
    d. An impression is a negative reproduction of the patient's dental arch. Once this impression is poured with a gypsum product, the end result will be a positive reproduction of the dental arch.

99. The impression automix system can be used for all but which of the following?
    d. A putty wash system is prepared in a totally different process than the syringe tray technique for which the automix system has been designed.

100. The process by which the resin material is changed from a pliable state to a hardened restoration is known as:
    a. A light-cured material does not harden until it has been exposed to a curing light. This allows a more flexible working time.

101. If humidity is high while mixing a final impression material, the setting time may be:
    a. High humidity will cause the impression material to set more quickly; thus, the setting time is decreased.

102. Select two terms that describe the purpose and consistency of a dental cement used for the seating of a temporary crown.
    d. The seating of a temporary crown requires a cement base that is of luting or primary consistency, which strings for about an inch. The purpose of seating the crown is for temporary cementation.

103. An onlay is a cast restoration that differs from an inlay in that the onlay includes the _____, _____, and some or all of the _____ to avoid future fracture.
    a. An inlay involves the occlusal surface and one or more proximal walls but does not provide for protection of cuspal surfaces. An onlay includes the complete occlusal table, both proximal surfaces, and some or all of the cusp surfaces to avoid future fracture.

104. A resin bonded bridge is commonly referred to as a _____.
    b. The Maryland bridge requires a conservative preparation designed for a resin-retained bridge that requires a bonding procedure.

105. When surgical retraction is performed rather than using chemical gingival retraction, the procedure is referred to as _____.
    b. Electrosurgery, using a special electric tip, is a common method of performing gingival retraction. This technique quickly cuts away the excess tissue and controls the bleeding.

106. Which of the following instruments is used to trim soft tissue during an oral surgery procedure?
    c. Surgical scissors are used to trim soft tissue. Suture scissors are designed to only cut suture material. A surgical curette is used after extractions to scrape the interior of the socket to remove abscesses or diseased tissue. A scalpel is used to make a precise incision into soft tissue.

107. The eating disorder that can easily be recognized in the dental office by severe wear on the lingual surface of the teeth caused by stomach acid from repeated vomiting is:
    a. Bulimia is an eating disorder that is characterized by binge eating and self-induced vomiting. The stomach acid from vomiting results in severe wear on the lingual surface of the teeth.

108. Inflammation of the supporting tissues of the teeth that begins with _____ can progress into the connective tissue and alveolar bone that supports the teeth and become _____.
    c. Gingivitis is the first stage of periodontitis. Unless this condition is arrested, the inflammation progresses into the periodontium and develops into periodontitis.

109. The dentist retires to another state and closes the practice. The entire staff is released from employment and the records remain in the office, but the patients are not notified of the dentist's retirement. Failure to notify the patients of the changes in the practice is called:

b. A dentist has an obligation to inform the patients of any change in the practice ownership. If the dentist fails to notify the patients of the changes in the practice, the dentist is guilty of abandoning the patients.

110. The MyPyramid, formerly known as the Food Guide Pyramid, is an outline of what to eat each day. The food group represented by the second smallest section on the pyramid is:

b. The second smallest food group segment on the MyPyramid is meat and beans. The widths are a general guide, not exact proportions.

111. _____ are found mainly in fruits, grains, and vegetables and _____ are found in processed foods such as jelly, bread, crackers, and cookies.

c. Complex carbohydrates are found mainly in fruits, grains, and vegetables, while simple sugars are found in processed foods such as donuts, jelly, bread, and cookies. Simple sugars are absorbed first; the complex sugars must be processed before they can be absorbed into the intestinal tract.

112. The patient's record indicates that the status of the gingival tissue is bulbous, flattened, punched-out, and cratered. This statement describes:

b. Gingival contour is described using terms such as *bulbous, flattened, punched-out,* or *cratered.* A different set of terms is used to describe the color, texture, and consistency of the gingival.

113. Supragingival calculus is found on the _____ of the teeth, above the margin of the _____.

b. Supragingival calculus is found on the clinical crowns of the teeth, above the margin of the gingiva. It is readily visible as a yellowish-white deposit that may darken over time.

114. Subgingival calculus occurs _____ the gingival margin and can be _____ in color due to subgingival bleeding.

d. Subgingival calculus forms on root surfaces below the gingival margin and can extend into the periodontal pockets. It can be dark green or black.

115. Which are examples of local risk factors for periodontal disease?

b. The conditions such as overhanging restorations, orthodontic appliances, and removable partial dentures are all conditions within the oral cavity that can contribute to periodontal disease if not properly cared for.

116. Which of the following is *not* a component of a clinical record?

d. The recall card is a separate record or database from the clinical chart. It is based on this record or database that patients are notified of their next recall visit.

117. Which of the following records is considered a vital record?

a. Records are categorized according to their importance in the office. The patient's clinical chart is considered a vital record, which without its availability the patient history and treatment would not be available.

118. Which member of the dental team is legally required to report suspected child abuse?
  b. The dentist is the only member of the dental team legally required to report suspected child abuse, although all members of the team have a moral responsibility to report suspected abuse to the dentist.

119. The dentist informs you that a patient will need three appointments to complete a three-unit bridge. These appointments will likely be to:
  a. The appointment schedule to seat a bridge includes the preparation, the try on of the components, and then the final cementation appointment.

120. The administrative assistant has failed to maintain the recall system for the past four months. Which is likely to occur?
  a. The recall system is the lifeline of the practice. Unless patients are routinely recalled to the dental office for a preventive prophylaxis, the lack of follow-up treatment will cause decreased productivity.

Radiation Health and Safety

1. Label the solutions used in an automatic film processor.
  b. From left to right the solutions in an automatic film processor are (1) developing solution, (2) fixing solution, (3) water wash.

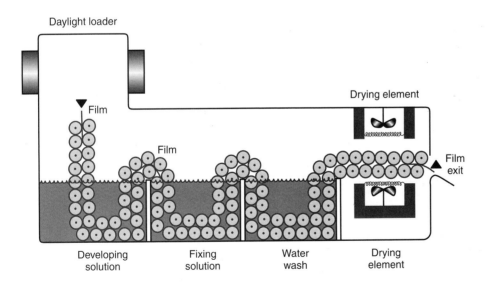

2. What is the landmark indicated by the arrows?
  b. This landmark is the incisive foramen, which is an opening or a hole in the bone located at the midline of the anterior portion of the hard palate directly posterior to the maxillary central incisors; it appears radiolucent.

3. What is the landmark circled on the radiograph?
  b. This is the lingual foramen. It is an opening or a hole in the bone located on the internal surface of the mandible near the midline; it is surrounded by the genial tubercles and appears radiolucent.

4. A bitewing film shows the _____ of both the _____ and _____.
  c. A bitewing film shows the crowns of both the maxilla and the mandible.

5. _____ is an example of a patient protection technique used before x-ray exposure.
  b. Proper prescribing of radiographs is an example of a patient protection technique because it limits the patient's exposure to radiation. The professional judgment of the dentist is used to determine the number, type, and frequency of dental radiographs. Every patient's dental condition is different, and therefore every patient must be evaluated for dental radiographs on an individual basis.

6. Which of the following is the recommended size of the beam at the patient's face?
  a. Federal regulations require that the diameter of the collimated x-ray beam be restricted to 2.75 inches at the patient's skin.

7. The _____ is an extension of the x-ray tubehead and is used to direct the x-ray beam.
  b. The positioning indicating device (PID) is an open-ended lead-lined cylinder extending from the opening of the metal housing of the tubehead; it aims and shapes the x-ray beam (also called the cone).

8. The collimator:
  b. The collimator is a diaphragm, usually lead, used to restrict the size and shape of the x-ray beam.

9. Which of the following types of PIDs do *not* produce scatter radiation?
  d. Neither the rectangular nor cylinder type PIDs allow the escape of scatter radiation. However, the pointed cone, which was originally designed as a user-friendly aiming device, with the tip of the cone indicating the position of the central ray does permit scatter radiation.

10. The thyroid collar:
  d. The thyroid collar is recommended for all intraoral films and is designed to be a separate shield or is part of the lead apron.

11. After the lead apron is used it should be:
  d. Once the lead apron has been used, it must be disinfected and hung up or laid on a rounded bar. It should never be folded, as it will crack and permanent damage will make it ineffective.

12. The_____ film provides a wide view of the maxilla and mandible.
  c. The panoramic film is an extraoral radiograph that is designed to provide a wide view of the maxilla and mandible on a single film

13. _____ film can be used in cassettes.
  c. An extraoral radiographic examination provides inspection of large areas of the skull or jaws using film placed in a cassette outside the mouth. The cassette is a light-tight device that holds the film and intensifying screens.

14. Which device is used to assist in the position of the PID in relation to the tooth and film?
  c. An assortment of beam alignment devices is available to enable the operator to align the beam properly in relation to the tooth and film.

15. Rules of radiation protection for the operator include all of the following *except* _____.
  c. Distance recommendations indicate that the radiographer must stand at least 6 feet away from the x-ray tubehead during x-ray exposure or a protective barrier must be used.

16. In order to increase the contrast on a radiograph, one should _____ the kilovoltage peak.
  a. Contrast refers to how sharply dark and light areas are differentiated or separated on a film. When low kilovoltage peak settings are used, a high contrast film will result.

17. Which of the following statements is *true* about duplicating films?
   d. The duplicating film has a direct positive emulsion; therefore, if more film density is needed (darker film), the exposure time is shortened. This is the opposite of time requirements for exposing dental film to x-rays.

18. Radiation caries is most often seen on teeth:
   c. During radiation treatment of head and neck cancer, the patient may have xerostomia if the field of radiation is in line with the mandible, maxilla, and salivary glands. The altered quantity and quality of saliva make the patient more susceptible to rampant type of caries at the cervical sites.

19. A tissue that lies within the primary dental beam and is very radiosensitive is the _____.
   b. When evaluating the effects of radiation on tissues and organs, the cornea is considered a high sensitivity organ.

20. When x-ray exposure time is increased, there is _____ density of the radiograph.
   a. An increase in exposure time increases film density by increasing the total number of x-rays that reach the film surface.

21. The overall blackness or darkness of a film is _____.
   b. Density is the overall darkness or blackness of a film. An adjustment in kilovoltage peak results in a change in the density of a dental radiograph.

22. Which of these would appear radiopaque on a radiograph?
   c. The enamel is the outermost radiopaque layer of the crown of the tooth. The portion of a processed radiograph that is light or white is one that resists the passage of the x-ray beam and limits the amount of x-rays that reach the film.

23. If the radiographic processing time is too long, the film will appear _____.
   a. A film that has been processed in the developer for too long will appear dark.

24. The hardening agent in processing fixer is(are):
   c. There are four basic ingredients in the fixer solution: fixing agent, preservative, hardening agent, and acidifier. The hardening agent in the fixer is composed of potassium alum.

25. Failure to add replenisher as needed each day to an automatic processor will result in:
   b. Processing solution levels in the automatic processor must be checked at the beginning of each day and replenished as necessary. Failure to add replenisher results in exhausted solutions and nondiagnostic radiographs.

26. X-ray film can be removed from the fixer after _____ minutes for a wet reading and _____.
   b. Following manufacturer's directions requires that x-ray film can be removed from the fixer after 3 minutes for a wet reading and then returned to the fixer for the remainder of processing.

27. What is the optimum development time and temperature for radiographic films using manual processing?
   d. According to manufacturer's directions, the optimum development time and temperature for radiographic films using manual processing is 68 degrees for 5 minutes.

28. An overdeveloped film may be caused by which of the following?
   c. Too long a time in the developer during processing will result in an overdeveloped film.

29. In a dental practice where many HIV-positive patients are treated, the film rollers in the automatic processor should be:
   d. Using standard precautions, all processing equipment is maintained in the usual accepted manner for all patients.

30. When using the bisecting technique, the imaginary angle that is bisected is formed between the long axis of the tooth and the:
    c. In the bisecting technique, the film must be placed along the lingual surface of the tooth. At the point where the film contacts the tooth, the plane of the film and the long axis of the tooth form an angle. The dental radiographer must visualize a plane that divides in half, or bisects, the angle formed by the film and the long axis of the tooth. This plane is termed the *imaginary bisector*. This bisector creates two equal angles and provides a common side for the two imaginary equal triangles.

31. For patients with bilateral mandibular impactions, the right and left lateral oblique techniques have been replaced by:
    c. Panoramic films are the choice for visualizing both right and left mandibular impactions.

32. In TMJ radiography, it is preferable to take films in the _____ position(s).
    c. The TMJ tomography is used to examine the TMJ. It is a radiographic technique used to show structures located within a selected plane of tissue while blurring structures outside the selected plane. It can be used in an open and closed format.

33. The computer used for digital imaging:
    b. Computers used in the modern dental office can be used interchangeably for digital imaging as well as routine office functions.

34. What is the problem with this radiograph?
    c. If film is developed at an elevated temperature and then placed in a cold water bath, the sudden change causes the swollen emulsion to shrink rapidly and gives the image a wrinkled appearance called *reticulation*.

35. On intraoral radiographs, when the patient's right is on your right, this is called _____ mounting.
    d. When radiographs are mounted so that the patient's right is on your right, this is type of mounting is from a lingual perspective.

36. A periapical lesion would appear _____ __ on processed radiographs.
    b. A periapical lesion located at the apex of a tooth will appear radiolucent or dark.

37. Radiographically, the appearance of a "dry socket" resembles:
    a. The appearance of a "dry socket" resembles a normal healing socket as there are no other distinguishing features of this condition radiographically.

38. Personnel monitoring of radiation exposure:
    b. The amount of x-radiation that reaches the body of the dental radiographer can be measured through the use of a personnel-monitoring device known as a film badge. The radiographer wears it for a specified time and the badge is returned to the service company, which in turn provides to the dental office an exposure report for each radiographer.

39. When a patient expresses concern about the need for radiographs, which of the following statements should be avoided?
    d. The dental radiographer must be prepared to explain exactly how patients are protected before, during, and after x-ray exposure. The patient must also be informed that only x-rays prescribed by the doctor will be exposed and that each patient is treated based on their individual needs and not as a routine procedure.

40. The _____ radiograph provides a view that shows the tooth crown, root tip, and surrounding structures of a specific area.
    b. The periapical radiograph provides a view that shows the tooth crown, root tip, and surrounding structures of a specific area and is widely used in diagnostic procedures.

41. Which type of PID would be most effective in reducing patient exposure?
    d. The 16-inch rectangular PID provides the most effective reduction of x-radiation during routine patient exposures.

42. Which of the following conditions exist on this film?
  b. This view indicates open contacts between the maxillary premolars as evidenced by the dark spaces between these teeth.

43. What is the landmark indicated by the arrows?
  a. The radiolucent area identified in this view is the mental foramen, an opening or a hole in bone located on the external surface of the mandible in the region of the mandibular premolars.

44. What is the landmark indicated by the arrows?
  d. The tubelike passageway through bone in the mandible that appears radiolucent is the mandibular canal.

45. What is the landmark indicated by the arrows?
  c. The radiolucent area in this film is the floor of the maxillary sinus, which is one of a paired cavity or compartment of bone located within the maxilla.

46. A _____ is defined as a marked prominence or projection of bone.
  c. A process is defined as a marked prominence of bone; it appears radiopaque.

47. The sensitivity of a film to radiation exposure is _____.
  b. Film speed is defined as the sensitivity of a film to radiation exposure.

48. Inherent filtration in the dental x-ray tubehead:
  a. Inherent filtration takes place when the primary beam passes through the glass window of the x-ray tube, the insulating oil, and the tubehead seal. Inherent filtration alone does not meet the standards regulated by state and federal law. Therefore, added filtration is required.

49. Which is *not* one of the three basic types of (PIDs)?
  d. Position indicating devices are provided in rectangular, conical, and round shapes but not in a square shape.

50. At what age should a full adult series be considered for a child?
  c. After age 9, the full adult series is taken, with the narrow adult film being used where necessary. These age guidelines are flexible and depend on the growth and development of the child.

51. The _____ radiographic view shows the crowns of teeth of both arches on one film.
  a. Bitewing radiographs show the crowns of the teeth of both arches on one film. These films are useful in examining the interproximal tooth surfaces.

52. Commercially available barrier envelopes:
  b. Barrier envelopes that fit over intraoral films can be used to protect the film packets from saliva and minimize contamination after exposure of the film.

53. Occlusal film is so named because it is _____ than periapical or bitewing film and the patient _____ the entire film.
  b. The occlusal film is used for examination of large areas of the maxilla or mandible. It is so named because the film is larger and the patient occludes or bites on the film.

54. Exposed films should _____ dried and then placed in a _____ for transport to the darkroom for processing.
  d. Exposed films should be dried and then placed in a disposable container for transport to the darkroom for processing.

55. The _____ radiograph is the film of choice for the evaluation of apical lesions.
  b. The periapical radiograph is the film of choice for evaluation of apical lesions as it shows all of the tooth including the crown, root, and apical region.

56. The radiograph most commonly exposed for an orthodontic patient is the:
  c. The cephalometric radiograph demonstrates the bones of the face and skull as well as the soft tissue profile of the face and is used by the orthodontist in diagnosis.

57. The minimum number of exposures for a full mouth survey of radiographs would be:
  b. The minimum number of films used in a full mouth survey would be 14. More films may be taken dependent on the doctor's prescription for the individual patient.

58. Developer solution has a(n) _____ pH, and fixer solution has a(n) _____ pH.
  c. According to the chemical composition of processing solutions, the developer solution has a basic pH and fixer solution has an acidic pH.

59. The purpose of a hardening agent is to harden and shrink the:
  d. The hardening agent shrinks and hardens the gelatin in the film emulsion.

60. The purpose of the fixing agent is to remove all _____ from the film emulsion.
  a. The fixing agent is made of sodium thiosulfate; ammonium thiosulfate functions to remove all unexposed undeveloped silver halide crystals from the emulsion.

61. The film emulsion is hardened during which of the following stages of the development process?
  c. It is during the fixing process that the film emulsion is hardened, using potassium alum as the hardening agent to shrink and harden the gelatin in the emulsion.

62. A stepwedge will reveal that radiographs taken at a higher kilovoltage peak will have _____ versus radiographs taken at a lower kilovoltage peak.
  a. A stepwedge is a device constructed of layered aluminum steps used to demonstrate film densities and contrast scales. It will reveal that radiographs taken at a higher kilovoltage peak will have long scale contrast versus radiographs taken at a lower kilovoltage peak.

63. A radiograph that has _____ is said to have low contrast.
  c. A film with many shades of gray has low contrast and may be difficult to use in a diagnosis.

64. Which of the following would appear the most radiolucent on a radiograph?
  c. The pulp cavity consists of the pulp chamber and pulp canals. It contains blood vessels, nerves, and lymphatics and appears relatively radiolucent on a dental radiograph.

65. Which of the following would appear most radiopaque?
  b. Amalgam is a common restorative material used in dentistry and is the most radiopaque of the substances listed in this question.

66. Label the orientation planes.
  The correct labels are 1, coronal; 2, sagittal; 3, transverse.

67. What is the landmark indicated by the arrows?
  c. The internal oblique ridge is a linear prominence of bone located on the internal surface of the mandible that extends downward and forward from the ramus. On a periapical radiograph, the internal oblique ridge appears as a radiopaque band that extends downward and forward from the ramus.

68. What is the landmark indicated by the arrows?
  b. The pulp cavity appears relatively radiolucent on a dental radiograph.

69. In this panoramic radiograph, which of the following statements is *true?*
  c. From this radiograph, it is evident that the permanent maxillary canines are malpositioned.

70. If you were mounting this film and the raised embossed dot was facing you, this film would be a _____ premolar view.
    b. When using labial mounting, all the raised dots face the viewer, and in this method the viewer is looking at the radiographs as if you were looking directly at the patient. In that case, this would be a maxillary left premolar view.

71. When mounting bitewing radiographs, mount them with the curve of Spee directed _____ toward the distal.
    a. The occlusal plane as it goes distally curves upward in what is called the curve of Spee.

72. Most tooth roots curve toward the _____.
    b. When looking at the anatomy of the teeth, it is evident that most roots curve toward the distal.

73. If you were mounting this film and the raised embossed dot was facing you, this film would be a _____ molar view.
    d. When using labial mounting, all the raised dots face the viewer, and in this method the viewer is looking at the radiographs as if you were looking directly at the patient. In that case, this film is a mandibular left molar view.

74. If you were mounting this film and the raised embossed dot was facing you, this film would be a _____ molar view.
    b. When using labial mounting, all the raised dots face the viewer, and in this method, the viewer is looking at the radiographs as if you were looking directly at the patient. In that case, this film is a maxillary left molar view.

75. Incorrect vertical angulation can result in an image that is:
    d. Incorrect vertical angulation can result in an image that is either foreshortened or elongated due to either increased or decreased vertical angulation.

76. Because of the curvature of the arch, the optimal number of bitewings is _____.
    b. Four bitewing radiographs are common procedure due to the curvature of the arch: two premolar and two molar views.

77. A two-film packet requires _____ exposure time as a one-film packet.
    a. The same amount of exposure time is used when a two-film packet is required for patient exposure.

78. The identification dot is used to:
    a. The use of the identification dot helps to determine film orientation as either lingual or labial orientation.

79. In a film packet, the thin lead foil sheet is positioned _____.
    b. The lead foil sheet is positioned behind the film to shield the film from scattered radiation.

80. Which of the following is a beam alignment device?
    d. A precision film holder will aid in beam alignment. The other devices are not used in beam alignment but may be used in film holding.

81. The _____ allows for the positioning of the tubehead.
    c. The extension arm of the x-ray machine is the part of the x-ray machine that suspends the x-ray tubehead and houses the electrical wires that extend from the control panel to the tubehead; its mobile arm helps in positioning the tubehead.

82. The acronym for the permitted lifetime accumulated dose is _____.
    c. The maximum accumulated dose (MAD) is the maximum radiation dose that may be received by persons who are occupationally exposed to radiation.

83. A _____ aids in stabilizing the film in the patient's mouth.
    c. A film holder may be of varying designs, but its primary function is to stabilize the film in the patient's mouth.

84. To test the automatic film processor, _____ in the automatic processor.
    d. Each day, two test films should be processed in the automatic processor. Unwrap two unexposed films, expose one to light, and then process both films. The results of the automatic processor test films can then be interpreted.

85. Which of the following may *not* be a radiographer?
    d. The primary role of the dental laboratory technician does not include exposing dental radiographs.

86. The time interval between radiographic examinations for children should be:
    d. As with all patients, the time interval and the number of radiographs prescribed for children should be based on individual needs of the child.

87. A patient with periodontal disease will likely require _____ radiographic examinations than a patient with a healthy periodontium.
    b. To follow the advancement of the periodontal disease of a patient, it may be required that the patient have more frequent radiographs than the patient with a healthy periodontium.

88. Prior to radiation exposure for a minor, informed consent:
    b. Consent for radiographs must be obtained from a parent or legal guardian. Legally, it cannot be obtained from another person.

89. To avoid occupation exposure to radiation, which is the most critical for a dental radiographer?
    d. Safe practice during radiographic exposure first requires that the radiographer avoid exposure to the primary beam.

90. The _____ radiation received and the ___the dose rate, the shorter is the latent period.
    d. The more radiation received and the faster the dose rate, the shorter will be the latent period. The latent period can be defined as the time that elapses between exposure to ionizing radiation and the appearance of observable clinical signs.

91. Which of the following changes will increase x-ray beam intensity?
    d. As x-rays travel away from their source of origin, the intensity of the beam lessens. Unless a corresponding change is made in one of the exposure factors (kilovoltage peak, milliamperage), the intensity of the x-ray beam is reduced as the distance increases.

92. The quantity of x-rays produced is controlled by _____.
    d. Milliamperage controls the penetrating power of the x-ray beam by controlling the number of electrons produced in the x-ray tube and the number of x-rays produced. Higher milliampere settings produce a beam with more energy, increasing the intensity of the x-ray beam.

93. What is the error in this film?
    b. Fixer spots are indicated in this film. This could occur during manual processing.

94. What is the error in this film?
    a. Scratch marks are evident on this film. This occurs when the soft emulsion is removed from the film by sharp objects. This is more common in manual processing when handling films on racks.

95. What is the error in this film?
    b. This film has limited diagnostic value as it is elongated and the apical region of the teeth are not present.

96. What is the manual processing error in this film?
   c. Developer cut off, the clear area on the film occurs during manual processing when the developer solution is too low in the tank and the exposed films are not completely immersed in the developing solution.

97. If the dot is facing the operator, this film shows the _____ region.
   d. When using labial mounting, all the raised dots face the viewer, and in this method the viewer is looking at the radiographs as if you were looking directly at the patient. In that case, this would be a mandibular left molar view.

98. This film is an example of a _____ radiograph.
   c. This is an occlusal radiograph showing the mandibular arch.

99. Which of the marked areas is the nasal septum?
   a. The nasal septum is shown in A; B is the nasal cavity, and C is the floor of the nasal cavity.

100. Which of the marked areas is the floor of the nasal cavity?
   c. The nasal septum is shown in A; B is the nasal cavity, and C is the floor of the nasal cavity.

Infection Control

1. If you opt not to receive a hepatitis B vaccination, you will be required to sign a(n):
   c. If an employee initially declines the vaccination but at a later date opts to have the vaccine and is still covered under the standard, the employer must provide the vaccine at no cost to the employee.

2. All dental professionals must use surgical masks and protective eyewear to protect the eyes and face:
   c. In accordance with the OSHA Bloodborne Pathogens Standard, masks and protective eyewear are to be worn whenever splashes, spray, spatter, or droplets of blood or saliva may be generated and eye, nose, or mouth contamination may occur.

3. All dental assistants involved in the direct provision of patient care must undergo routine training in:
   a. The OSHA standard requires that employers shall ensure that all employees with occupational exposure participate in a training program on the hazards associated with body fluids, protective measures to ensure safe practice, as well as hazard communications processes.

4. _____ occurs from a person previously contracting a disease and then recovers.
   a. When a microorganism invades the body, it usually activates a special host defense system. Once this system is activated, it attempts to prevent serious harm from the microorganism and may provide protection against future invasions of the body by that same microorganism. This process is call naturally acquired immunity.

5. _____ immunity occurs when a vaccination is administered and the body forms antibodies in response to the vaccine.
   b. Artificial immunity involves being immunized or vaccinated against a specific disease so that the body forms antibodies in response to the vaccine.

6. A latent infection is best exemplified by which of the following?
   b. A cold sore is a type of latent infection as it is quiet and inactive without manifesting itself until a period of incubation occurs.

7. Which of the following exemplifies an acute infection?

c. An acute infection is one that has a rapid onset, severe symptoms, and a short course. The common cold is an example of such an infection.

8. Microorganisms that produce disease in humans are known as:

b. A pathogen is a microorganism capable of causing disease in its host.

9. A(n) _____ is a person who is unable to resist infection by a pathogen.

b. A susceptible host is an individual who has little resistance to a disease or has become immune to the disease.

10. An infection that occurs when the body's ability to resist diseases is weakened is a(n):

d. An opportunistic disease is one that will occur in the body when the person is unable to resist the infection or when the infection is given the opportunity.

11. A disease that can be transmitted in some way from one host to another is a(n):

d. *Infectious, contagious,* and *communicable* are all terms that refer to diseases that can be transmitted from one host to another.

12. The transmission of a disease through the skin, as with cuts or punctures, is _____ transmission.

b. Parenteral transmission of an infection refers to a mode of transmission that occurs through punctures or cuts in the skin.

13. Which of the following would be considered the best method for determining whether there is proper sterilization function by a sterilizer?

c. Biological monitoring or spore testing provides the main guarantee of sterilization accomplished by a sterilizer.

14. When the assistant prepares a package of hazardous infectious waste for disposal, which of the following statements is true?

a. Following recommended procedures, hazardous infectious waste should be placed in closable, leak-proof containers or bags that are color coded or labeled appropriately.

15. Protective eyewear should have _____.

c. Eyewear worn by the dental health care worker should have side shields to protect from aerosols and spatter.

16. Exam gloves used during dental treatment can be made of:

d. Latex or vinyl is the primary material of which acceptable examination gloves are made.

17. Infectious or regulated waste (biohazard) include all of the following *except* _____.

d. X-ray wrappers do not fall into the category of infectious or regulated waste. These items are not pathogenic waste, nor are they likely to be saturated with blood or other potentially infectious materials (OPIM).

18. Which of the following statements is *not* true as they apply to the use of overgloves?

d. Overgloves are not acceptable alone as a hand barrier in nonsurgical procedures. These gloves are used over the examination gloves when the assistant leaves the room or wants to prevent contamination of an area with the examination gloves.

19. During which of the following procedures would you use sterile surgical gloves?

d. A mandibular resection is an invasive surgical procedure and would require the use of surgical gloves.

20. Which of the following statements is *not* an appropriate action for postexposure medical evaluation and follow-up?
    a. After the exposure incident, the employer must make immediately available to the exposed employee a medical evaluation performed by a licensed physician or other licensed health care professional at no cost to the employee.

21. Which of the following is a cause of sterilization failure?
    c. A closed container prevents direct contact with the sterilizer agent.

22. To prevent contamination of surfaces, which of the following techniques should be used?
    b. Applying covers after the surfaces become contaminated is a waste of money and time because the contaminated surfaces will have to be precleaned and disinfected when the patient leaves. The covers should be placed before the surfaces become contaminated and the cover should be carefully removed without touching the underlying surface. Covering surfaces is intended to replace precleaning and disinfecting between patients.

23. An emergency action plan may be communicated orally if the workplace has fewer than _____ employees.
    d. According to the Fire Safety Standard of OSHA, an employer must review with each employee on initial assignment all parts of the fire safety plan that the employee must know to protect coworkers and patients in the event of an emergency. For offices with fewer than 10 employees, the plan may be communicated orally, and the employer is not required to maintain a written plan.

24. What is the maximum volume that a single container of alcohol-based hand rub solution placed within a dental treatment room can legally have?
    c. The American Society of Healthcare Engineering has issued a set of rules that include the placement of alcohol-based hand rubs. One of these rules states that single containers installed in the dental treatment room should not exceed a maximum capacity of 2.0 L of alcohol-based rub solutions in gel/liquid form.

25. All of the following surfaces *except* one may need to be cleaned and disinfected before each patient appointment. Which one is the exception?
    b. Floors must be cleaned routinely but not after each patient. All of the other surfaces come into direct contact with patient care and must be cleaned and disinfected after each patient.

26. A tip for protecting dental instruments includes all of the following *except* _____.
    d. Instruments are only dried prior to dry heat or chemical vapor sterilization to avoid corrosion aspects in these sterilizers.

27. Protective eyewear should have:
    d. Protective eyewear must have side shields to prevent eyes from being contaminated from aerosols.

28. The costs associated with hepatitis B vaccines of at risk employees are:
    b. In accordance with the OSHA Bloodborne Pathogens Standard, the vaccine must be made available to the employee at no cost to the employee.

29. Bacteria that make acids are called _____.
c. Bacteria that produce acids during growth are called acidogenic. Acidogenic and aciduric bacteria are important in the initiation and progression of dental caries in the patient's mouth.

30. Bacteria that die in the presence of oxygen are known as _____.
b. Nonaerobic or anaerobic bacteria cannot tolerate oxygen and grow only in its absence.

31. When an assistant transfers a microbe from one patient to his or her hand and then to another patient's mouth, this transmission is referred to as _____.
b. The mode of transmission where the disease results from injuries with contaminated sharps or from contact with contaminated instruments, equipment, or surfaces is known as indirect contact.

32. A(n) _____ is a protein manufactured in the body that binds to and destroys microbes and other antigens.
b. An antibody is a protein produced in response to an antigen that is capable of binding specifically to that antigen.

33. The strength of an organism in its ability to produce disease is:
a. Virulence is the degree of pathogenicity possessed by an organism to produce disease.

34. Another name for airborne transmission is:
c. *Airborne* and *droplet* are synonymous terms in that they cause disease through small liquid droplets.

35. Pathogens that are carried in the blood and body fluids of infected individuals and that can be transmitted to others are referred to as:
a. Bloodborne pathogens are disease-producing microorganisms that are spread by contact with blood or other body fluids from an infected person.

36. Recommendations concerning gloves would fall under which of the following categories of infection control practices that directly relate to dental radiography procedures?
b. Personal protective equipment includes gloves, eyewear, and masks that are worn during routine clinical treatment to protect the dental health care worker.

37. Protective clothing:
d. In accordance with OSHA recommendations, protective clothing must prevent skin and mucous membrane exposure when contact with blood or other bodily fluids is anticipated.

38. Which of the following is an infectious disease?
c. When tissue is damaged by microorganisms, the process is referred to as an infectious disease.

39. The substance in a vaccine that stimulates an immune response is called an _____.
c. Artificial immunity occurs when a person is immunized or vaccinated against a specific disease. The person is inoculated with an antigen such as dead microorganisms, weakened microorganisms, the antigenic part of a microorganism, or an inactivated toxin that will not cause disease or damage to the body but will stimulate the immune system.

40. How does HIV cause AIDS?
d. HIV is capable of destroying the body's defense against disease and lowers the immune system's ability to resist the disease.

41. The risk of getting HIV as a dental assistant is:
d. The CDC reports that the risk of HIV disease transmission from dental patients to members of the dental team is low.

42. When using medical latex or vinyl gloves, _____.
b. Nonsterile gloves are recommended for routine dental care and nonsurgical procedures. Sterile gloves would be used in surgical or invasive procedures.

43. ___ is defined as the absence of pathogens, or disease-causing microorganisms.
    d. The absence of infection or infectious materials or agents is known as the state of asepsis.

44. Antiseptic is:
    b. Antiseptics are chemical agents that can be used on external tissues to safely destroy microorganisms or to inhibit their growth.

45. A disease arising from within the body that is caused by opportunistic microorganisms already present in the body is referred to as a(n) _____ infection.
    c. Endogenous infections occur from the inside from opportunistic microorganisms that are already present in the body.

46. Which of the following agents is *not* tuberculocidal?
    b. Quaternary ammonium compounds are categorized as low-level disinfectants and none are tuberculocidal.

47. When can a liquid sterilant/high-level disinfectant achieve sterilization?
    b. High-level disinfectants can achieve sterilization when the solution is used only for longer exposure times in accordance with manufacturer's directions.

48. Which of the following may be used for surface disinfectant in the dental office?
    a. Most iodophors are intermediate-level disinfectants and can be used for surfaces in the treatment room. They do have a slightly corrosive effect to some metals and may cause a light staining if used repeatedly.

49. Sterilizers such as autoclaves are preset to reach a maximum steam temperature of ___ degrees Fahrenheit and a pressure of ___ pounds per square inch (psi).
    c. Most manufacturers today preset the autoclave for steam under pressure sterilization to reach 250° F and pressure of 15 to 30 psi.

50. When using the _____ method of sterilization, instruments must be absolutely dry or they will rust.
    a. Each instrument placed in the chemical vapor sterilizer must be dried before processing in this sterilizer or the residual water remaining on the instruments can override the rust-free process.

51. Which of the following is considered to be a semicritical instrument in radiography?
    d. The x-ray film holding device is considered a semicritical instrument, although if it is used intraorally, it would not likely come in contact with blood.

52. The stage of an infectious disease when the patient's symptoms begin to subside is called _____.
    d. The convalescent stage of an infectious disease occurs as the patient's symptoms begin to subside, the number of microorganisms may be declining, and the harmful microbial products are destroyed rapidly as the body seeks to combat the disease.

53. This method of sterilization requires good ventilation.
    c. Unsaturated chemical vapor sterilization requires that good ventilation be available in the sterilization area.

54. Which of the following microbes are well known for causing periodic recurrences after the initial infection?
    c. The human herpes virus is known for causing periodic recurrences after the initial infection. Human herpes virus type 1 may cause infections of the mouth, skin, eyes, and genitals of those persons who have depressed immune systems.

55. Which government agency requires employers to protect their employees from exposure to blood and saliva at work?
    d. The OSHA Bloodborne Pathogens Standard is the most important infection control law in dentistry to protect the dental health care workers.

56. If a thorough job of cleaning or sterilizing reusable hand instruments is *not* accomplished, this will contribute to which pathway of cross-contamination in the office?
    b. Patient-to-patient disease transmission is an indirect transfer of disease through improperly prepared instruments, handpieces and attachments, treatment room surfaces, and hands.

57. When using this method of sterilization, the exposure time varies as to whether the instruments are wrapped or unwrapped.
    d. According to the manufacturer's directions for flash sterilization, the exposure time will vary dependent on whether the instruments are wrapped or unwrapped.

58. From the list below, select the best procedure for caring for orthodontic wire.
    c. Orthodontic wire is defined as a sharp and is placed in the sharps container at the end of use.

59. From the list below, select the best procedure for caring for a pair of crown and collar scissors.
    a. With sharp edges on the crown and collar scissors, the most efficient method of sterilization would be to place the scissors in a protective emulsion prior to placing in steam under pressure.

60. From the list below, select the best procedure for caring for a pair of surgical suction tips.
    b. A surgical suction tip is generally made of metal and does not have any sharp edges. Therefore, it can be safely and efficiently placed in steam under pressure sterilization without the need to be placed in emulsion first.

61. Which of the following is the recommended scheme for immunization against hepatitis B?
    a. The recommended scheme for immunization against hepatitis B for the dental health care worker is 0, 1, and 6 months.

62. From the list below, select the best procedure for caring for a mandrel.
    b. A mandrel may be placed in steam under pressure without emulsion.

63. The intent of handwashing is to remove:
    a. The microorganisms of transient skin flora contaminate the hands during the touching of or other exposure to contaminated surfaces. These flora serve as a source of disease spread because it can contain just about any pathogenic microorganism. Transient skin flora can be reduced or removed in some cases by routine handwashing because they remain primarily on the outer layers of the skin.

64. From the list below, select the best procedure for caring for a pair of protective glasses.
    c. Protective eyewear cannot be subjected to heat and therefore must be immersed in a cold chemical agent.

65. What is the active agent in hand rubs acceptable for use in dental offices?
    d. The agent in hand rubs used in the dental office is alcohol. It is used without water and without rinsing.

66. Which type of sterilization used in the dental office requires the longest processing time?
    c. Dry heat takes longer to sterilize than does steam under pressure or chemical vapor; it takes 1 hour at 320° F to 370° F depending on the type of sterilizer.

67. Immersion in a chemical liquid sterilant requires at least ___ hour(s) of contact time for sterilization to occur.
    b. Immersion sterilization/high-level disinfectant requires an extended contact time of 10 hours. This time may vary according to the manufacturer.

68. Instruments have been in a liquid sterilant for 2 hours. The assistant adds another batch of instruments. Which of the following statements addresses this situation?
    d. Retiming must begin again when the second batch of instruments has been added to the original instruments that were immersed. The status of the original instruments has been altered, thus the retiming.

69. The ideal instrument processing area should be:
    b. The ideal processing area for instruments would be dedicated solely to instrument processing.

70. What should the work flow pattern be for processing contaminated instruments?
    b. When instruments are processed, the work flow pattern starts at the dirty area, proceeds to the clean area, then to the sterile area, and finally to the storage area.

71. Which of the following methods of precleaning dental instruments should be avoided?
    c. Hand scrubbing is not a safe method for precleaning instruments. Instrument washing machines, rinsing in a holding solution, and ultrasonic cleaning are the most efficient and safe modes of precleaning and cleaning instruments.

72. Which statement is *not* true about an ultrasonic cleaner?
    c. The ultrasonic cleaner is used for cleaning instruments only. It does not disinfect or sterilize instruments.

73. After instruments have completed the cleaning cycle of the ultrasonic cleaner, they should be:
    b. Before proceeding with disinfection or sterilization after cleaning in the ultrasonic cleaner, the instruments must be rinsed with clear water.

74. The last of the PPEs to be put on before patient treatment begins is(are):
    c. For maximum efficiency and safe practice, while donning the PPEs, the last to be placed are the gloves.

75. Heavy utility gloves should be used:
    d. Heavy utility gloves are worn when processing contaminated instruments.

76. Which of the following statements is *not* true as it relates to the use of glutaraldehyde as an immersion disinfectant/sterilant?
    b. Glutaraldehyde is toxic and it is recommended that it be used in a well-ventilated area; when not in use, the jar or bottle should be covered.

77. The sterilization process is best described as being:
    b. The sterilization is sporicidal in that it destroys all microorganisms including high number of bacterial spores.

78. The process that kills disease-causing microorganisms, but not necessarily all microbial life, is defined as:
    c. Disinfection destroys vegetative bacteria, some fungi, and some viruses; it does not destroy *Mycobacterium tuberculosis* var *bovis*.

79. The best way to determine that sterilization has actually occurred is to use:
    b. Biologic monitoring provides the most efficient guarantee of sterilization.

80. Low-level disinfection can be used for:
    c. Low-level disinfection can be used for housekeeping surfaces such as floors, walls, and noncritical surfaces without visible blood; as well as clinical contact surfaces.

81. Patient care instruments are categorized into various classifications. Into which classification would instruments such as impression trays, dental mouth mirror, and amalgam condenser be placed?
    b. Impression trays, the dental mouth mirror, and the amalgam condenser are considered to be semicritical instruments.

82. Which of the following does *not* minimize the amount of dental aerosols and spatter generated during treatment?
    a. The amount of aerosols and spatter generated during dental treatment is not reduced by preprocedural mouth rinses. However, studies have shown that a mouth rinse with a long-lasting antimicrobial agent can reduce the level of oral microorganisms for up to 5 hours.

83. Which of the following microbes are *not* killed by intermediate-level disinfection?
    a. Intermediate-level disinfectants destroy vegetative bacteria, most fungi, and most viruses as well as inactivates *Mycobacterium tuberculosis* var *bovis* but does not kill bacterial spores.

84. Which of the following is *not* a recommended PPE for cleaning and disinfecting a dental treatment room?
    c. For safe practice, latex gloves are not the PPE of choice for cleaning and disinfecting a dental treatment room and its equipment.

85. OSHA requires a *minimum* of training of dental personnel in all of the following areas *except* _____.
    c. The OSHA standard does not require specialty safety standards as part of dental personnel training.

86. Which of the following statements is *true* as it relates to the environmental infection control in a clinical area?
    b. The use of carpet and cloth-upholstered furnishings inhibits the ease of caring for these surfaces as it is not possible to disinfect them efficiently.

87. The Organization for Safety and Asepsis Procedures identifies the classification of clinical touch surfaces to include which of the following?
    b. Clinical touch surfaces include light handles, dental unit controls, and chair switches, all items that are commonly touched during routine clinical treatment.

88. Chemicals that destroy or inactivate most species of pathogenic microorganisms on inanimate surfaces are called:
    a. Disinfectants are used to destroy or inactivate most pathogenic microorganisms on inanimate surfaces such as countertops and flat cupboard surfaces.

89. Who determines the hazards of a chemical?
    c. The dental manufacturer is responsible for determining the hazards of a chemical and must provide an MSDS for each product sent to the dental office.

90. When a denture is being sent to a commercial laboratory, it should _____.
    d. When a denture, other prosthesis, or an impression is sent to a commercial laboratory, it should be disinfected before being sent out and then again after being received back from the laboratory.

91. A victim who feels the effects of a chemical spill immediately, with symptoms of dizziness, headache, nausea, and vomiting, is experiencing:
    b. When a person experiences an acute chemical toxicity, he or she will feel the effects immediately and will experience dizziness, headache, nausea, and vomiting.

92. _____ is considered regulated waste and requires special disposal.
    a. Teeth and other waste tissues are considered potentially infectious, and thus their disposal should be regulated.

93. The office safety supervisor should check the contents of the emergency kit to determine that the contents are in place and within the expiration date _____.
    b. First aid and emergency kits should be labeled and stored in an area easily accessible to the dental staff but out of sight of patients. This kit should be checked each month to ensure currency.

94. Which of the following statements is *true* concerning cleaning and disinfection of the dental unit and environmental surfaces?
    a. When cleaning the dental unit and other bulky equipment in the treatment room, it is necessary to use an intermediate level disinfectant.

95. All waste containers that hold potentially infectious materials must:
    b. In accordance with OSHA regulations, all potentially infectious waste must be labeled with the biohazard symbol.

96. The OSHA Hazard Communications Standard requires employers to do all *except* _____.
    d. The OSHA Hazard Communications Standard does not require employees to submit to an annual hair test.

97. A DHCW transfers a small amount of cavity medication into a smaller container for use on a patient at chairside. A new label must be placed on that container if:
    b. When it is necessary to transfer a small amount of cavity medication from a large container into a smaller one, the new container must be labeled if it is not used up at the end of an 8-hour workday.

98. When recapping the needle, the dental assistant should use any of the following methods *except* _____.
    d. A two-handed scoop method is not an acceptable method of recapping a needle. It promotes potential accidents and can result in a needle stick injury.

99. During which phase is it likely the microbes begin to multiply and form a spreading film or layer on the tubing walls of dental unit hosing?
    b. The accumulation stage is when microbes begin to multiply and start to form a spreading film or layer on the tubing walls.

100. The ADA, OSAP, and CDC recommend that the dental assistant:
    b. Various agencies, including ADA, OSAP, and CDC, recommend that the dental assistant flush the dental unit waterlines for 20 to 30 seconds each morning and after each patient.

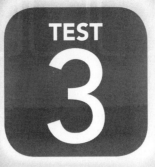

TEST

3

General Chairside, Radiation Health and Safety, and Infection Control

General Chairside

Directions: Select the response that best answers each of the following questions. Only one response is correct.

1. In the universal lettering system for primary teeth, which letter stands for the maxillary left second molar?
   a. K
   b. J
   c. T
   d. C

2. The type of caries that occurs on the occlusal surfaces or the buccal and lingual grooves of posterior teeth is(are) _____.
   a. root surface caries
   b. smooth surface caries
   c. pit and fissure caries
   d. secondary caries

3. Which of the following is *not* one of the components of the ABCDs of basic life support?
   a. access
   b. breathing
   c. circulation
   d. defibrillation

4. What does this charting symbol indicate?
   a. gold crown
   b. stainless steel crown
   c. missing tooth
   d. post and core

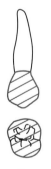

5. Which surgical procedure describes a hemisection?
   a. removal of the apical portion of the root
   b. removal of diseased tissue through scraping with a curette
   c. removal of one or more roots of a multirooted tooth without removing the crown
   d. removal of the root and crown by cutting through each lengthwise

6. What does this charting symbol indicate?
   a. root canal
   b. missing tooth
   c. impacted tooth
   d. rotated tooth

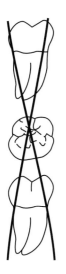

7. What does this charting symbol indicate?
   a. full crown
   b. implant
   c. root canal
   d. bonded veneer

8. The respiration rate for an adult who has just participated in an aerobic activity might be:
   a. 10 to 20
   b. 18 to 30
   c. 20 to 40
   d. 80 to 110

9. What does this charting symbol indicate?
   a. implant
   b. fracture
   c. diastema
   d. root canal

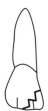

10. Using Black's classification of cavities, a lesion on the cervical third of a tooth is considered a Class _____ restoration or cavity.
   a. I
   b. II
   c. III
   d. V

11. The abbreviation used in the progress notes or chart to indicate a mesioocclusodistal restoration with a buccal extension would be:
   a. MeOcDiL
   b. LDOM
   c. MODB
   d. DOML

12. When working with anesthetic needles, the _____ the gauge number, the thicker is the needle.
   a. larger
   b. smaller

13. The hard palate is recorded in the _____ impression.
   a. mandibular
   b. maxillary

14. The tooth-numbering system that uses a two-digit tooth recording system with the first digit indicating the quadrant and the second digit indicating the tooth within the quadrant, with numbering from the midline to the posterior, is referred to as the:
    a. Universal System
    b. Palmer Notation System
    c. Fédération Dentaire Internationale System
    d. Bracket Numbering System

15. Which of the following statements is *not* true as it relates to a patient's respiration?
    a. If a patient knows the breaths are being monitored, he or she will usually change the breathing pattern.
    b. For children and teenagers, the respiration rate is higher than that of an adult.
    c. A person's respiration normally is not noticeable unless he or she is having trouble taking a breath.
    d. Respirations are normally higher in counts per minute than the pulse rate.

16. The respiration pattern of a patient in a state of tachypnea has:
    a. a slow respiration rate
    b. excessively short, rapid breaths
    c. excessively long, rapid breaths
    d. a gurgling sound

17. The respirations of a patient who is hyperventilating will be exemplified by:
    a. a slow respiration rate
    b. excessively short, rapid breaths
    c. excessively long, rapid breaths
    d. a gurgling sound

18. A patient who displays symptoms of unconsciousness, increased body temperature, rapid heart beat, and increased blood pressure may be displaying symptoms of:
    a. a petit mal seizure
    b. a grand mal seizure
    c. hypoglycemia
    d. hyperglycemia

19. If a patient displays symptoms of hypoglycemia and is conscious, what is the first thing you should ask the patient?
    a. "What time did you awaken this morning?"
    b. "When did you last eat and did you take insulin?"
    c. "How many fingers do you see?" while holding up your fingers.
    d. "Did you bring some lunch?"

20. The MyPyramid is an outline of what to eat each day. The smallest segment of the pyramid represents:
    a. grains
    b. vegetables
    c. meats
    d. oils

21. Any food that contains sugars or other carbohydrates that can be metabolized by bacteria in plaque is described as being:
    a. sweet
    b. cariogenic
    c. composed of empty calories
    d. a complex carbohydrate

22. Organic substances that occur in plant and animal tissues are _____, and essential elements that are needed in small amounts to maintain health and function are _____.
    a. minerals, vitamins
    b. fat-soluble vitamins, water-soluble vitamins
    c. vitamins, minerals
    d. cholesterol, minerals

23. A horizontal or transverse plane divides the body into:
    a. superior and inferior portions
    b. dorsal and ventral portions
    c. anterior and posterior portions
    d. medial and lateral portions

24. Which of these instruments is a combination DE instrument used as an explorer and periodontal probe?
    a. shepherd's hook
    b. cowhorn explorer
    c. right angle explorer
    d. expro

25. The forceps are used in this portion of the clamp while placing the rubber dam. Ⓑ

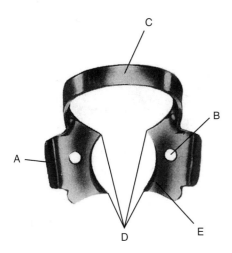

26. Which of the following statements is *false* as it relates to correct use of the HVE tip?
    a. When using a surgical suction tip, it may be necessary to flush it with water periodically.
    b. Use the thumb to nose or pen grasp according to the location of placement of the tip.
    c. All HVE tips are disposable.
    d. When placing the tip, the assistant should place the HVE tip first and then the operator should place the handpiece.

27. The water-to-powder ratio generally used for an adult maxillary impression is _____ measures of water, _____ scoops of powder.
    a. 3, 3
    b. 3, 2
    c. 3, 4
    d. 2, 2

28. High-volume evacuation provides all *except* _____ which of the following.
    a. increases the patient's desire to rinse
    b. decreases the patient's desire to rinse
    c. decreases the amount of aerosol emanating from the patient's mouth
    d. increases visibility

29. Which of the following statements is *not* a concept of four-handed dentistry?
    a. Place the patient in the supine position.
    b. The operator and assistant should be as close to the patient as possible.
    c. Use present tray setups with instruments placed in sequence of use.
    d. Use a wide winged patient chairback.

30. The _____ handpiece can operate both forward and backward and can be used with a variety of attachments.
    a. high-speed
    b. laboratory
    c. low-speed
    d. laser

31. When the Tofflemire matrix band retainer is used, which of the knobs or devices would be used to adjust the size or loop of the matrix band to fit around the tooth and loosen the band for removal?

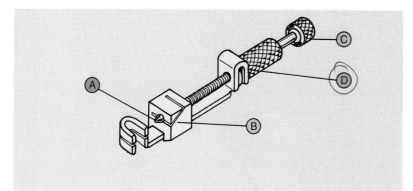

32. Which of the following instruments is a K style file?

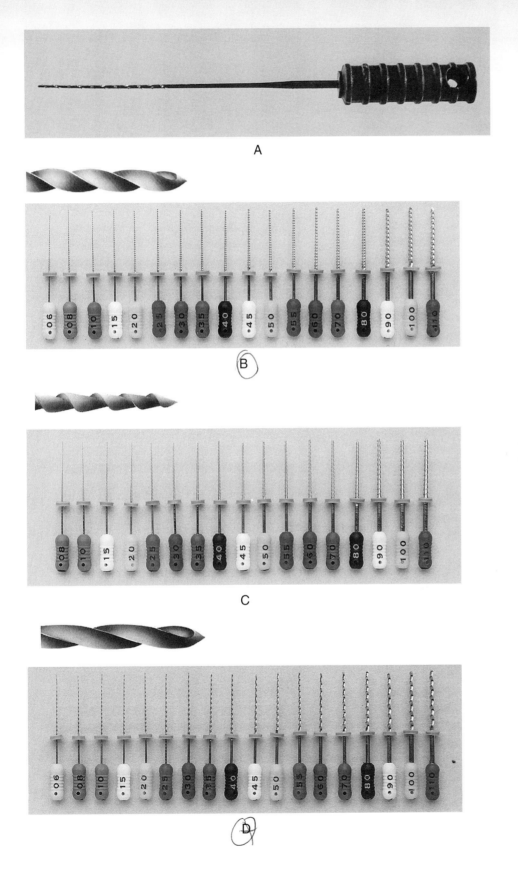

A

B

C

D

33. Which of the following instruments would be used to remove debris or granulation tissue from a surgical site?
    a. rongeur forceps
    b. surgical curette
    c. periodontal probe
    d. periosteal elevator

34. Which of the following statements is *true* when using a Tofflemire matrix band and retainer?
    a. The matrix retainer and wedge are both placed on the buccal.
    b. The matrix retainer is placed on the buccal and the wedge is placed from the lingual at the proximal surface involved.
    c. The matrix retainer is placed on the lingual and the wedge is placed from the buccal at the proximal surface involved.
    d. It is not necessary to use a wedge with a Tofflemire matrix band and retainer.

35. The dental team is completing an amalgam procedure on 4^MOD. Which of the following statements is *true*?
    a. One wedge and no smooth surface carvers would be used.
    b. Two wedges, smooth surface, and anatomical carvers would be used.
    c. There is no need to use a matrix band and retainer in this situation.
    d. There is no need to use wedges in this situation.

36. When a two-paste system is used for a composite material, the paste of either jar should not be cross-contaminated because:
    a. it will cause the material to harden
    b. it will prevent the material from hardening
    c. the translucency will be diminished
    d. polymerization will be delayed

37. Which the following statements is *false* as it relates to the acid etching of enamel for a composite restoration?
    a. The acid-etching agent forms a mechanical bond with the enamel.
    b. The acid-etching agent is flooded onto the surface and rubbed vigorously.
    c. The material is generally applied with special applicators provided by the manufacturer. ✓
    d. The acid-etching agent is rinsed from the tooth after recommended time to stop the etching process. ✓

38. When cleaning a dental handpiece, it is important to:
    a. follow the handpiece manufacturer's directions thoroughly
    b. follow the sterilizer manufacturer's directions thoroughly
    c. always lubricate the handpiece prior to sterilization
    d. always lubricate the handpiece after sterilization

39. Which of the following rotary instruments would cut faster and most efficiently?
    a. tungsten carbide bur
    b. stainless steel bur
    c. diamond stone
    d. green stone

40. Which classification(s) of motions should the dentist and the dental assistant eliminate to increase productivity and decrease stress and body fatigue?
    a. Class I — ~~wrist fig~~
    b. Class II — wrist & fingi
    c. Class III finger, wrist & elbows.
    d. Classes IV and V

41. Which of the following conditions is *not* a potential medical contraindication to nitrous oxide?
    a. nasal obstruction
    b. emphysema and multiple sclerosis
    c. emotional instability
    d. age

42. What substance is added to a local anesthetic agent to slow down the intake of the agent and increase the duration of action?
    a. sodium chloride
    b. a vasoconstrictor
    c. an amide
    d. an ester

43. The type of anesthesia achieved by injecting the anesthetic solution directly into the tissue at the site of the dental procedure is known as _____.
    a. inferior alveolar nerve block anesthesia
    b. block anesthesia
    c. infiltration anesthesia
    d. incisive nerve block

44. General anesthesia is most safely administered in a(n):
    a. general dentist's office
    b. oral surgeon's office
    c. hospital ✓
    d. periodontist's office

45. An orthodontic positioner is designed to:
    a. move the teeth
    b. retain the teeth in their desired position
    c. reposition the teeth during orthodontic treatment
    d. both a and c

46. Which of these would *not* be a choice of instrument to place gingival retraction cord?
    a. explorer
    b. cord packing instrument
    c. blunt end of a plastic instrument

47. From the photograph below, what is the procedure for which this tray would be used?
    a. preparation for a cast restoration
    b. cementation of a cast restoration
    c. placement of brackets
    d. placement of separators

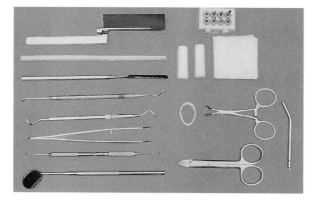

48. The instruments shown below from left to right are:
    a. three-pronged pliers, posterior band remover, ligature pin, ligature cutter
    b. Howe pliers, wire bending pliers, ligature tying pliers
    c. bird beak pliers, contouring pliers, Weingart utility pliers
    d. bird beak pliers, Howe pliers, wire bending pliers

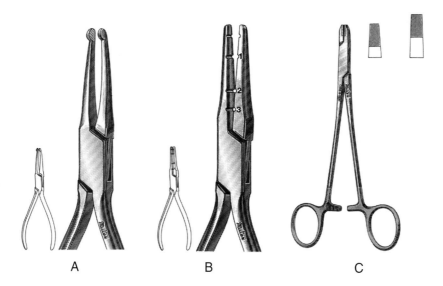

A   B   C

49. To control bleeding after a surgical procedure, the patient should be instructed to do all of the following *except* _____.
    a. Bite on a folded sterile 2 × 2 gauze for at least 30 minutes after the procedure is completed.
    b. If bleeding continues and does not stop, call the dental office.
    c. Restrict strenuous work or physical activity for that day.
    d. Rinse vigorously after 6 hours.

50. What is the endodontic test in which the dentist applies pressure to the mucosa above the apex of the root and notes any sensitivity or swelling?
    a. percussion
    b. palpation
    c. cold
    d. electric pulp vitality

51. The process by which the living jawbone naturally grows around the implanted dental supports is known as:
    a. subperiosteal integration
    b. transosteal implantation
    c. osseointegration
    d. osseus transintegration

52. The treatment used as an attempt to save the pulp and encourage the formation of dentin at the site of the injury is a(n):
    a. pulp capping
    b. pulpectomy
    c. apicoectomy
    d. pulpotomy

53. The removal of the coronal portion of an exposed vital pulp is a(n):
    a. pulpectomy
    b. pulpotomy
    c. apicoectomy
    d. root resection

54. The instrument used to adapt and condense gutta-percha points into the canal during endodontic treatment is:
    a. Gates Glidden bur
    b. spreader/plugger
    c. endodontic spoon excavator
    d. broach

55. The surgical removal of diseased gingival tissues is called:
    a. gingivoplasty
    b. gingivectomy
    c. osteoplasty
    d. osteoectomy

56. A(n) _____ is a dentist with a license in the specialty of dentistry who provides restoration and replacement of natural teeth and supporting structures.
   a. endodontist
   b. periodontist
   c. orthodontist
   d. prosthodontist

57. Periodontal pocket depth is charted at _____ points on each tooth during a baseline charting procedure.
   a. two
   b. four
   c. six
   d. eight

58. A periodontal pocket marker is similar in design to a _____.
   a. thumb forceps
   b. cotton pliers
   c. Gracey scaler
   d. periodontal probe

59. A(n) _____ is an additive bone surgery that includes the reshaping and contouring of the bone.
   a. ostectomy
   b. osteoplasty
   c. gingivoplasty
   d. apicoectomy

60. From the instruments shown below, select the periosteal elevator.

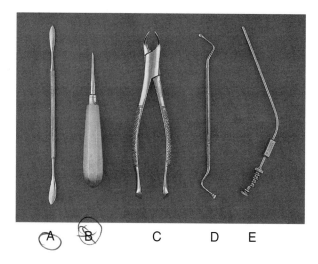

   A   B   C   D   E

61. Using Black's classification of cavities, a pit and fissure lesion on the occlusal surface of molars and premolars is considered a Class _____ cavity.
  a. I
  b. II
  c. III
  d. V

62. Using Black's classification of cavities, a pit lesion on the buccal surface of molars and premolars is considered a Class _____ restoration or cavity.
  a. I
  b. II
  c. III
  d. V

63. The more fixed attachment of the muscle that is usually the end attached to the more rigid part of the skeleton is the:
  a. origin
  b. insertion
  c. contraction
  d. infraction

64. Which of the following teeth would *not* be found in the deciduous dentition?
  a. lateral incisor
  b. cuspid
  c. second premolar
  d. second molar

65. A red line is used on this tooth. What does this charting symbol indicate?
  a. missing
  b. to be extracted
  c. root canal
  d. impacted

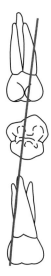

66. What does this charting symbol indicate?
   a. recurrent decay
   b. amalgam
   c. sealant
   d. missing

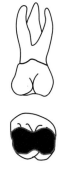
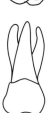

67. On a cephalometric analysis, the abbreviation Na stands for:
   a. anterior nasal spine
   b. gnathion
   c. nasion
   d. menton

68. Which orthodontic pliers are used in fitting bands for fixed or removable appliances?
   a. bird beak pliers
   b. contouring pliers
   c. posterior band remover pliers
   d. Howe (110) pliers

69. If the charting conditions indicate that there is a furcation involvement, some type of symbol will be placed:
   a. at the apical area of the tooth
   b. on the occlusal surface of the tooth
   c. at the area between two or more root branches
   d. at the cervical region

70. A reproduction of an individual tooth on which a wax pattern may be constructed for a cast crown is a(n):
   a. die
   b. model
   c. cast
   d. impression

71. Which of the following materials would *not* be used to take a final impression for the creation of a prosthetic device?
    a. silicone
    b. polysiloxane
    c. alginate hydrocolloid
    d. agar hydrocolloid

72. A porcelain fused to metal crown would be designed so the porcelain would always be on the _____ surface.
    a. lingual
    b. buccal/facial
    c. mesial
    d. distal

73. A glass ionomer material may be used for all of the following *except* a(n):
    a. restorative material
    b. liner
    c. luting agent
    d. obtundant

74. If the room temperature and humidity are very low while mixing a final impression material, the setting time may be:
    a. decreased
    b. increased

75. A porcelain fused to metal crown is being seated. The assistant will mix the cement to a _____ or _____ consistency.
    a. base, secondary
    b. cementation, secondary
    c. base, primary
    d. cementation, primary

76. A posterior tooth with a deep preparation may require a base that is designed to prepare pulpal defense by functioning as a(n):
    a. final restoration
    b. protective base
    c. insulating base
    d. sedative base

77. A patient has a fractured amalgam on 29DO. Time in the doctor's schedule does not permit placement of a permanent restoration. Which of the following statements is *correct* as to the type of dental cement and the consistency that would be used in this clinical situation?
    a. temporary cement to a secondary consistency
    b. final cement to a secondary consistency
    c. temporary cement to a primary consistency
    d. final cement to a primary consistency

78. An alginate impression has been taken to prepare a set of diagnostic models. Which of the following statements is *false* as it relates to handling the impression? Alginate impressions _____.
   a. should be stored for as short a period as possible
   c. shrink when stored in air with low humidity
   b. expand when stored in water
   d. can be stored in 100% relative humidity without serious dimensional changes for up to 24 hours

79. IRM (intermediate restorative material) is used primarily for:
   a. final restorative for primary molars
   b. provisional restoration
   c. cementing crowns bridges and onlays
   d. seating an implant

80. Dry mouth is also known as _____.
   a. periodontal disease
   b. blastomia
   c. xerostomia
   d. glossitis

81. _____ is more prominent in older adults who have experienced gingival recession.
   a. Interproximal dental decay
   b. Cervical caries
   c. Incisal caries
   d. Generalized dental decay

82. Which food can be compared to a reversible hydrocolloid?
   a. potato chips
   b. salad dressing
   c. ice cream
   d. ketchup

83. Which of the following could *not* be suggested as an intervention for the prevention of dental caries?
   a. fluoride
   b. antibacterial therapy
   c. decreased ingestion of carbohydrates
   d. chewing mints

84. A caries risk assessment test is used to _____.
   a. determine the number of mutans streptococci and lactobacilli count present in the saliva
   b. determine the amount of fermentable carbohydrate present in the saliva
   c. determine the salinity of the saliva
   d. determine the level of salivary immunity

85. Inflammation of the supporting tissues of the teeth that begins with _____ can progress into the connective tissue and alveolar bone that supports the teeth and become _____.
   a. gingivitis, glossitis
   b. periodontitis, gingivitis
   c. gingivitis, periodontitis
   d. gingivitis, gangrene

86. A dietary food analysis includes a diary of everything a patient consumes for:
  a. 24 hours
  b. 72 hours
  c. 1 week
  d. 1 month

87. The MyPyramid is an outline of what to eat each day. Which of the following statements is *true* regarding a food pyramid:
  a. All food pyramids include a base formed of dairy products.
  b. The largest portion of a vegetarian food pyramid is dairy products.
  c. Recent research has provided a food pyramid for a vegetarian diet.
  d. The food pyramid is a myth.

88. From the photograph below, which of these instruments is a T-ball burnisher?

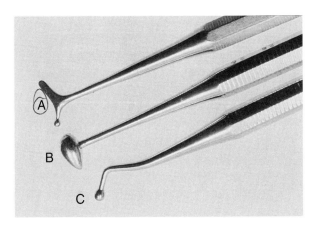

89. The patient's record indicates that the status of the gingiva is bulbous, flattened, punched-out, and cratered. This statement describes the gingival _____:
  a. color
  b. contour
  c. consistency
  d. surface texture

90. Supragingival calculus is found on the _____ of the teeth, above the margin of the _____.
  a. cervical region, periodontal ligament
  b. clinical crowns, gingiva
  c. anatomical crowns, periodontal ligament
  d. cervical margins, apex

91. Subgingival calculus occurs _____ the gingival margin and can be _____ in color due to subgingival bleeding.
    a. above, yellow
    b. below, yellow
    c. above, red
    d. below, black

92. All of the following are types of restorations *except* _____.
    a. Class I
    b. Class X
    c. Class IV
    d. Class V

93. _____ sealants _____ require mixing as they cure when they are exposed to UV light.
    a. Chemically cured, do
    b. Light cured, do
    c. Chemically cured, do not
    d. Light cured, do not

94. When adjusting a crown after cementation, the dentist most likely would use a _____.
    a. diamond bur
    b. FG bur
    c. stone
    d. RA bur

95. The procedure that is done to remove subgingival calculus and to remove necrotic tissue from the periodontal pocket is referred to as a _____:
    a. root planing
    b. prophylaxis
    c. coronal polishing
    d. gingival curettage

96. The _____ provides rapid calculus removal and reduces operator hand fatigue.
    a. Gracey scaler
    b. sickle scaler
    c. ultrasonic scaler
    d. curette scaler

97. A(n) _____ procedure is performed to remove defects and to restore normal contours in the bone.
    a. gingivectomy
    b. gingivoplasty
    c. osseous surgery
    d. frenectomy

98. Which of the following is *not* a measurement used in constructing a complete denture?
    a. protrusion
    b. lateral excursion
    c. centric relation
    d. reversion

99. When transferring patient records from the office to another site, the administrative assistant must do all *except* which of the following?
    a. Obtain consent from the patient or legal representative.
    b. Retain the original record in the office.
    c. Transfer the entire record.
    d. Copy the radiographs and retain the originals.

100. A new filing system for clinical charts is to be installed in your office. Which of the following filing systems would be most efficient?
    a. open files with colored filing labels with alpha and numeric codes
    b. vertical files with tab-top labels
    c. vertical files with closed-end folders
    d. lateral files with closed-end folders

101. If an administrative assistant chooses to transmit a transaction about a patient electronically, under which act does this task fall?
    a. ADA
    b. HHS
    c. HIPAA
    d. NIOSHA

102. A message about a serious illness or allergy should be noted in which manner on the clinical record?
    a. on the outside of the record in large bright color
    b. inside the record in a discreet but obvious manner such as a small brightly colored label
    c. in large print on the lower-right edge of the outside of the record
    d. in large print inside the record

103. The group responsible for establishing regulations that govern the practice of dentistry within a state is the:
    a. American Dental Association
    b. Dental Assisting National Board
    c. Commission on Dental Accreditation
    d. Board of Dentistry

104. The act of doing something that a reasonably prudent person would not do or not doing something that a reasonably prudent person would do is:
    a. fraud
    b. abandonment
    c. negligence
    d. defamation of character

105. The universal retainer is also referred to as the _____ retainer.
    a. Tofflemire
    b. Matrix
    c. Black's
    d. extension

106. A clinical dental assistant is hired in the practice. The dentist indicates that this person is to place an intracoronal provisional restoration. The person knows how to perform the task but does not yet have the EFDA credential required to perform the specific intraoral task. What should you suggest to her when she asks you what she should do?
   a. Do what the dentist told her to do.
   b. Perform the task now but later tell the dentist that she does not have the appropriate credential.
   c. Inform the dentist that she does not yet have the appropriate credential to perform the task.
   d. Perform the task with the self-assurance that she will soon have her credential.

107. The Good Samaritan Law offers incentives for health care providers to provide medical assistance to injured persons without the fear of potential litigation *except* under which of the following circumstances?
   a. protection for a negligent health care provider who is being compensated for services
   b. immunity for acts performed by a person who renders care in an emergency situation
   c. when the provider is solely interested in providing care in a safe manner, with no intent to do bodily harm

108. The objectives of good appointment book management include all *except* which of the following?
   a. maximize productivity
   b. reduce staff tension
   c. maintain concern for the patient needs
   d. allow for maximum downtime

109. In reference to appointment management, prime time refers to:
   a. the time during which the dentist performs the most expensive type of treatment
   b. the time most frequently requested by patients
   c. the first 2 hours of the daily schedule
   d. midday appointment times

110. Which time of day is considered most appropriate when treating young children?
   a. just prior to naptime
   b. immediately following naptime
   c. early morning
   d. late in the day

111. What type of supply is a curing light used in a dental office?
   a. expendable
   b. nonexpendable
   c. capital
   d. variable

112. A patient has the following amalgam restorations: 29MO, 30^{MOD}, 31DO, and 32°. The fee for each surface is $115. What is the fee for services rendered?
   a. $320
   b. $420
   c. $880
   d. $920

113. Light curing:
   a. relies on ultraviolet light.
   b. is used to polymerize composite resin restorative material and composite resin cement.
   c. is used to polymerize silver dental amalgam.
   d. is called auto-polymerization.

114. The tip of the composite curing light should be held at an angle of __ degrees to the tooth.
   a. 10
   b. 25
   c. 45
   d. 90

115. Composite restorative materials are usually cured for __ seconds with the halogen curing light.
   a. 3
   b. 20
   c. 60
   d. 120

116. The removable denture prosthesis can be cleaned in the dental office by all of the methods listed below EXCEPT:
   a. immersion in an ultrasonic cleaner with a special denture cleaning solution.
   b. brushing with a denture brush.
   c. removing calculus with hand instruments.
   d. with routine prophylaxis instruments and brushes in the patient's mouth.

117. A broken removable denture prosthesis can be repaired:
   a. at home by the patient with an OTC kit.
   b. at home by the patient with superglue.
   c. in the office with cold-cured acrylic.
   d. in the office with light-cured composite.

118. _____ cement must be mixed on a glass slab.
   a. Zinc polycarboxylate
   b. Zinc oxide-eugenol
   c. Zinc phosphate
   d. Calcium hydroxide

119. Which of the following materials is recommended for polishing filled hybrid composites and resin restorations?
   a. silex and tin oxide
   b. aluminum oxide paste
   c. diamond polishing paste
   d. coarse polishing paste

120. A maxillary denture _____ have a full palate and a mandibular denture _____ have a full palate.
   a. will: will
   b. will: will not
   c. will not: will
   d. will not: will not

Radiation Health and Safety

Directions: Select the response that best answers each of the following questions. Only one response is correct.

1 The_____ film provides a view that shows the bony and soft tissue areas of the facial profile.
a. bitewing
b. periapical
c. panoramic
d. cephalometric

2. In digital radiography, the sensor replaces the _____.
a. x-ray beam
b. film processor
c. intraoral dental film
d. x-ray machine

3. Digital radiography requires _____ x-radiation conventional radiography because the sensor is _____ sensitive to x-rays than conventional film.
a. less, more
b. more, less
c. less, less
d. more, more

4. Examples of conditions resulting in smooth root resorption are _____ and _____.
a. infection, trauma
b. tumors, cysts

5. Who is the guardian of a patient's dental records?
a. the patient
b. the court
c. the dentist

6. The _____ radiograph is the film of choice for the intraoral examination of large areas of the upper or lower jaw.
a. occlusal
b. periapical
c. bitewing
d. panoramic

7. The _____ radiograph is the film of choice for the extraoral examination of the upper or lower jaw.
a. occlusal
b. periapical
c. bitewing
d. panoramic

8. A(n) _____ is a lesion characterized by a localized mass of granulation tissue around the apex of a nonvital tooth; appears radiolucent.
   a. pulp stone
   b. periapical granuloma
   c. amalgam tattoo

9. The most common cause of poor definition in a radiograph is _____,
   a. size of patient
   b. type of film used
   c. movement
   d. improper horizontal angulation

10. A film that has been fogged will have decreased:
    a. contrast
    b. density
    c. size
    d. life

11. Presently, the maximum permissible dose (MPD) for dental workers with ionizing radiation is _____.
    a. 2 rem/year
    b. 5 rem/year
    c. 10 rem/year
    d. 25 rem/year

12. Light leaks in a darkroom will cause:
    a. overdevelopment of the film
    b. underdevelopment of the film
    c. fogging of the film
    d. herringbone

13. The types of radiation interaction with patients include all of the following *except* _____.
    a. primary
    b. secondary
    c. tertiary
    d. scatter

14. If the radiographic processing time is too short, the film will appear _____.
    a. dark
    b. light
    c. clear
    d. fogged

15. Which is the correct sequence for processing x-ray film?
    a. rinse, develop, fix, rinse, dry
    b. develop, rinse, fix, rinse, dry
    c. fix, rinse, develop, rinse, dry
    d. develop, fix, dry

16. The developing agent in the developer solution is:
    a. hydroquinone and elon
    b. hydroquinone and sodium sulfite
    c. sodium sulfite and sodium carbonate
    d. elon and potassium bromide

17. An overdeveloped film may be caused by which of the following?
    a. inadequate development time
    b. solution that is too warm
    c. excessive development time
    d. concentrated developer solution

18. When using the bisecting techniques, the imaginary angle that is bisected is formed between the long axis of the tooth and the:
    a. long axis of the PID
    b. horizontal axis of the film
    c. long axis of the film
    d. horizontal axis of the tube head.

19. An application of tomography used in dentistry is:
    a. silography
    b. digital radiography
    c. scanning of the temporomandibular joint

20. _____ enables viewing of an area in three planes.
    a. Digital radiography
    b. Computed tomography
    c. Panoramic projection
    d. Cephalometric projection

21. What would a fluoride artifact look like on a radiograph?
    a. splotches on the radiograph
    b. black marks on the radiograph
    c. white spots on the radiograph
    d. multiple black linear streaks

22. On intraoral radiographs, when the patient's right is on your left, the identification dot on the film will be:
    a. facing you
    b. away from you

23. A completed root canal would appear _____ on processed radiographs.
    a. radiopaque
    b. radiolucent
    c. geometric
    d. poorly defined

24. Which of the following will appear radiopaque on a radiograph?
   a. periapical granuloma
   b. first-stage periapical cemental dysplasia
   c. periapical cyst
   d. cement base under a restoration

25. A supernumerary tooth in the midline is referred to as a(n):
   a. odontoform
   b. mesiodens
   c. enamel pearl
   d. pulp stone

26. Which of the following statements is *not* true about a bitewing radiograph?
   a. The film is placed in the mouth parallel to the crowns of both the upper and lower teeth.
   b. The film is stabilized when the patient bites on the bitewing tab or bitewing film holder.
   c. The central ray of the x-ray beam is directed through the contacts of the teeth, using a vertical angulation of +40.
   d. The bitewing radiograph is a method used to examine the interproximal surfaces of the teeth.

27. If a lead apron is folded after being used, it will _____ and _____.
   a. shred, mold
   b. crack, become ineffective
   c. gradually fall apart, become powdery
   d. crack, remain effective

28. The lead apron is:
   a. recommended for intraoral films
   b. not recommended for extraoral films
   c. an option; use is not mandated by any state or federal law
   d. used to protect the thyroid gland

29. Added filtration in the dental x-ray tubehead:
   a. refers to the placement of tungsten disks in the path of the x-ray beam between the collimator and the tubehead seal
   b. filters out shorter wavelength x-rays from the x-ray beam
   c. results in a lower energy beam
   d. results in a more penetrating useful beam

30. _____ is used to restrict the size and shape of the x-ray beam and to reduce patient exposure.
   a. Inherent filtration
   b. Added filtration
   c. Collimation
   d. PID

31. The radiopaque restoration on the first molar is:
   a. a composite restoration with an overhang on the mesial
   b. an amalgam restoration with an overhang on the mesial
   c. composite restoration with an overhang on the distal
   d. an amalgam restoration with an overhang on the distal

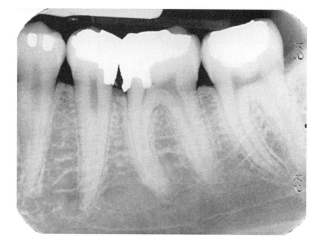

32. What is the landmark indicated by the arrows?
   a. coronoid process
   b. condyle
   c. internal oblique ridge
   d. mandibular canal

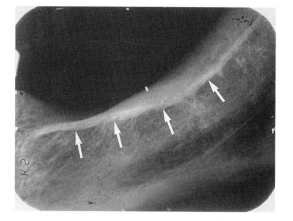

33. What is evident in this film?
   a. external resorption
   b. physiologic resorption
   c. internal resorption
   d. supernumerary tooth

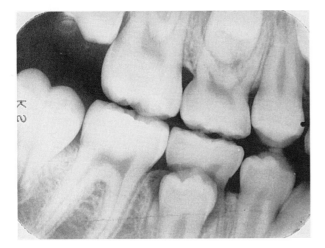

34. What is evident in this panoramic film?
   a. orthodontic appliances
   b. orthodontic bands
   c. metal framework for two partial dentures
   d. fused gold crowns

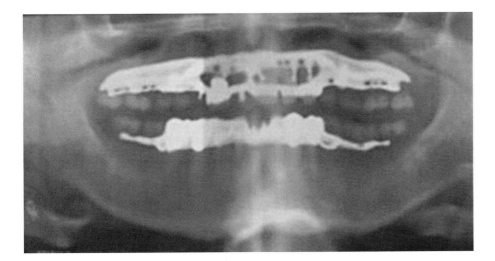

35. When the voltage is increased:
  a. electrons move from the anode to the cathode with more speed
  b. photons move from the anode to the cathode with more speed
  c. electrons move from the cathode to the anode with more speed
  d. photons move from the cathode to the anode with more speed

36. What is the landmark indicated by the arrows?
  a. coronoid process
  b. condyle
  c. internal oblique ridge
  d. zygomatic process of the maxilla

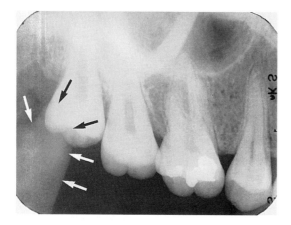

37. In which two lengths are PIDs typically available?
  a. 6 and 12 inches
  b. 12 and 24 inches
  c. 8 and 16 inches
  d. 12 and 16 inches

38. When a pregnant patient expresses concern about the need for radiographs, which of the following statements should be used?
  a. "The doctor told me to take these x-rays, so she would know best."
  b. "We use a lead apron and thyroid collar to protect your body from stray radiation, so don't worry!"
  c. "It is the rule of the office; otherwise, we can't treat you."
  d. "The doctor has ordered only the x-ray that is essential for your treatment today, and after you deliver we can take other x-rays as needed."

39. Which processing error results in the "herringbone effect"?
  a. collimator cutoff
  b. improper film placement
  c. film reversal
  d. overlapped films

40. What is the restoration on the mandibular first molar?
  a. gold crown
  b. stainless steel crown
  c. porcelain crown
  d. porcelain fused to metal crown

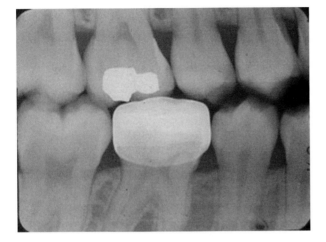

41. What is the restoration on the maxillary lateral incisor?
  a. porcelain fused to metal crown
  b. composite with radiopaque cement
  c. porcelain crown with radiopaque cement ✓
  d. stainless steel crown

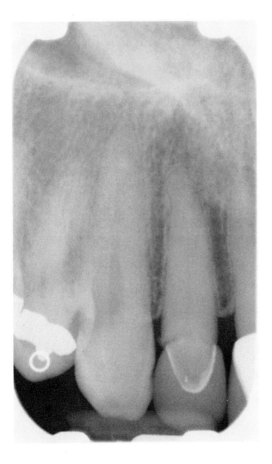

42. What is the restoration on the maxillary arch?
   a. five gold crowns
   b. porcelain fused to metal bridge
   c. three full crowns and two implants
   d. removable partial denture

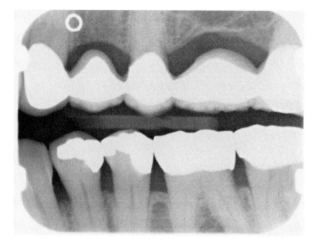

43. The "unsharpness," or blurring, that surrounds the edges of a radiographic image is the _____.
   a. photoelectric effect
   b. penumbra
   c. obliteration
   d. electromagnetism

44. _____ radiation is the penetrating x-ray beam that is produced at the target of the anode.
   a. Scatter
   b. Particulate
   c. Primary
   d. Leakage

45. _____ radiation is that form of radiation that is in the environment and includes cosmic and terrestrial radiation.
   a. Characteristic
   b. Scatter
   c. Braking
   d. Background

46. The median palatine suture appears _____ in a radiograph.
   a. radiolucent
   b. radiopaque

47. The film mounting method in which radiographs are placed in the film mouth with the depressed side of the identification dot facing the viewer is referred to as _____ mounting.
   a. lingual
   b. labial

48. The lead tubular device used to restrict the size and shape of the x-ray beam is the lead _____.
   a. glass housing
   b. switch
   c. collimator
   d. diaphragm

49. The _____ is a unit of measurement for dose equivalent; the SI unit equivalent to the rem.
   a. septa
   b. Sievert
   c. silver halide
   d. stepwedge

50. Regressive alteration of tooth structure that occurs within the crown or root of a tooth and appears radiolucent in a radiograph is _____.
   a. pathologic resorption
   b. internal resorption
   c. physiologic resorption
   d. external resorption

51. Which of these would *not* be a maxillary landmark for the maxilla in a panoramic view?
   a. styloid process
   b. external auditory meatus
   c. incisive canal
   d. mental foramen

52. Extraoral radiography will be used for all of the following *except* to _____.
   a. evaluate growth and development
   b. evaluate impacted teeth
   c. diagnose dental caries
   d. evaluate the extent of large lesions

53. If the _____ is not placed on the _____ during a panoramic radiographic exposure, a radiolucent shadow will be superimposed over the apices of the maxillary teeth.
   a. bite block, floor of the mouth
   b. tongue, roof of the mouth
   c. tongue, floor of the mouth
   d. bite block, roof of the mouth

54. A _____ lead apron is recommended for use during the exposure of a panoramic film.
   a. single-sided
   b. double-sided

55. _____ film is used in panoramic radiography.
   a. Screen
   b. Nonscreen
   c. Duplicating
   d. Periapical

56. Size 3 film is _____ and is used only for _____ images.
   a. smaller, periapical
   b. longer and narrower, bitewing
   c. wider and longer, bitewing
   d. longer and narrower, occlusal

57. The sizes available for bitewing film include:
   a. 0, 1, 2
   b. 0, 1, 2, 3
   c. 0, 1, 2, 3, 4
   d. 4 only

58. Size 0 film is most commonly used on:
   a. children
   b. average-sized adults
   c. large adults

59. The image shown in this projection is a:
   a. mandibular anterior periapical
   b. mandibular pediatric occlusal
   c. maxillary anterior periapical
   d. maxillary pediatric occlusal

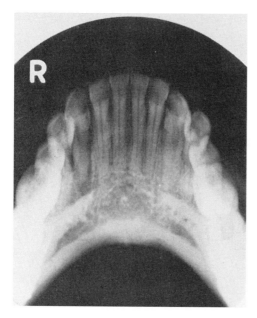

60. The image shown in this projection would require the patient be positioned with the mandibular arch:
   a. parallel to the floor
   b. at 45 degrees to the floor
   c. at right angles

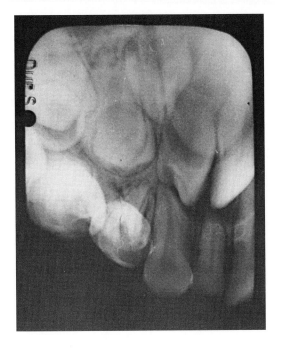

61. Which type of dentition best describes this radiograph?
   a. primary
   b. permanent
   c. mixed

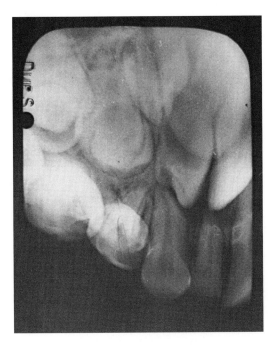

62. When exposing a molar bitewing, the following conditions should exist *except* _____.
   a. occlusal plane should be parallel to the floor.
   b. place a bitewing tab on the film
   c. center the film on the first molar
   d. direct the central beam through the contact areas of the molars

63. The image shown above the teeth in this projection is a(n):
   a. earring
   b. nose jewelry
   c. amalgam tattoo
   d. implant

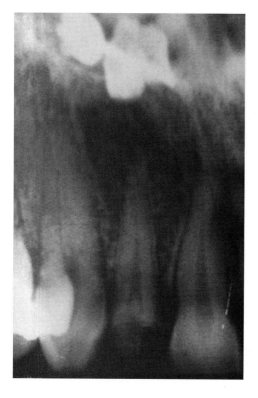

64. A severe carious lesion on a x-ray will:
   a. not penetrate the dentin
   b. extend through the enamel
   c. extend through the enamel and dentin and more than half the distance toward the pulp
   d. invade the dentin

65. Root caries involves:
   a. surfaces from the enamel through the pulp and into the root
   b. cementum and dentin only, not the enamel
   c. enamel and cementum
   d. cementum only

66. An anterior periapical film is oriented _____, and a posterior periapical film is oriented _____.
   a. vertically, horizontally
   b. horizontally, vertically
   c. vertically, vertically
   d. horizontally, horizontally

67. Which of the following is an advantage of digital radiography?
a. initial setup costs
b. image quality
c. increased speed of image viewing
d. legal issues

68. A concept of radiation protection that states that all exposure to radiation must be kept to a minimum is _____.
a. ALARA
b. Bremsstrahlung
c. Joule
d. Rogerian

69. The _____ governs the orientation of structures portrayed in two radiographs exposed at different angulations.
a. ALARA
b. buccal object rule
c. SLOB
d. right angle rule

70. The arrows indicate the _____ in this image.
a. nasal spine
b. median palatine suture
c. incisive foramen
d. superior foramina

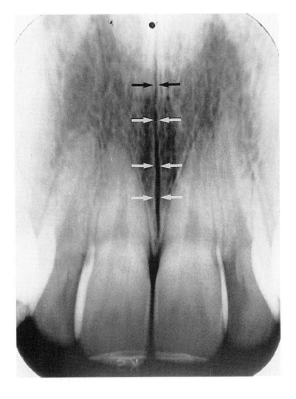

71. What is the error in this film?
a. cone cut
b. overlap
c. foreshortening
d. elongation

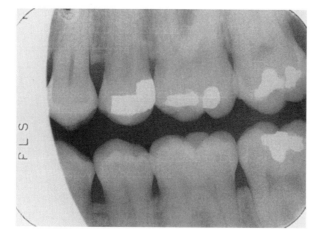

72. What is the error in exposure of this film?
a. incorrect horizontal angulation
b. incorrect vertical angulation
c. film placement
d. film size

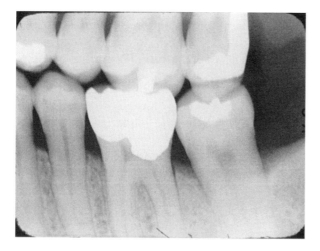

73. What is the error in exposure of this film?
   a. incorrect horizontal angulation
   b. incorrect vertical angulation
   c. film placement
   d. film size

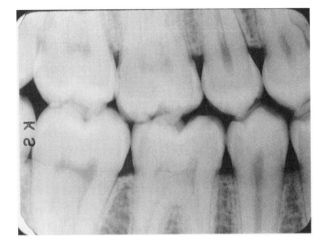

74. Which of the following definitions is *incorrect?*
   a. parallel: always separated by the same distance
   b. intersecting: to cut through
   c. right angle: formed by two parallel lines
   d. central ray: central portion of the beam

75. What do you respond when the patient asks who owns the dental radiographs?
   a. "The dentist, and if you want a copy, we will be glad to expose another set."
   b. "You do, and you may take them any time you want them."
   c. "The dentist, but this means you can request a copy of your dental radiographs or request that a copy be sent to the dentist of your choice."
   d. "The insurance company that paid for them."

76. A fogged film appears:
   a. gray and lacks detail and contrast
   b. black
   c. clear
   d. sharp and clear with good contrast

77. Static electricity appears as _____ on a film.
   a. black dots
   c. clear dots
   c. scratches
   d. black branching lines

78. Which of the following statements is *not* correct concerning the exposure sequence for periapical films?

 a. Anterior films are always exposed before posterior films.

 b. Either anterior or posterior films may be exposed first.

 c. In posterior quadrants, the premolar film is always exposed before the molar film.

 d. When exposing anterior films, work from the patient's right to left in the upper arch and then work from the left to right in the lower arch.

79. What piece of equipment is required to hold the film parallel to the long axis of the tooth in the paralleling technique?

 a. bitewing tab

 b. film holder

 c. cotton roll

 d. patient finger

80. What size film is used with the posterior XCP instrument?

 a. 0

 b. 1

 c. 2

 d. 4

81. What is the error in exposure of this film?

 a. foreshortening

 b. elongation

 c. cone cut

 d. film placement

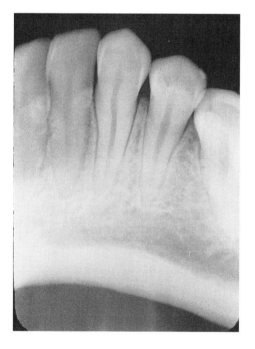

82. What person is responsible for the final and definitive interpretation of dental radiographs?
    a. dentist
    b. dental assistant
    c. dental hygienist
    d. dental insurance director

83. An explanation of what is viewed on a radiograph is _____, whereas the identification of a disease by examination and analysis is _____.
    a. knowledge, interpretation
    b. interpretation, diagnosis
    c. findings, diagnosis
    d. diagnosis, interpretation

84. The nucleus of an atom contains:
    a. protons
    b. neutrons
    c. protons and neutrons
    d. electrons

85. Which of the following statements is *true* regarding the direct theory of radiation injury?
    a. It involves absorption of an x-ray photon by water within a cell.
    b. It involves the combination of free radicals to form toxins.
    c. It involves a direct hit and absorption of an x-ray photon within a cell.
    d. Both a and b are true.

86. _____ regulate the manufacture and installation of dental x-ray equipment.
    a. The local government
    b. The municipality
    c. The state government
    d. The federal government

87. Which of the following statements is *true* regarding the placement of a film packet in the patient's mouth?
    a. The tube side of the film is white and has a raised bump in one corner; when placed in the mouth, the white side faces the teeth and the tubehead.
    b. The tube side of the film packet has a flap and is color coded; when placed in the mouth, the color-coded side of the packet must face the teeth and tubehead.
    c. The lead foil sheet is wrapped in black protective paper and is positioned in front of the film to shield the film from secondary radiation.
    d. A circle or dot that corresponds with the raised identification dot on the film appears on the lingual side of the film packet.

88. During formation of the latent image, irregularities in the lattice structure of the exposed crystal, known as the _____, attract silver atoms.
    a. protective layer
    b. emulsion
    c. sensitivity specks
    d. adhesive layer

89. Radiographs are a(n) _____ comprehensive patient care.
    a. vital component to
    b. adjunct to
    c. option for
    d. follow-up to

90. With faster F-speed film, a single intraoral film results in a surface skin exposure of _____ milliroentgens.
    a. 1.25
    b. 12.5
    c. 100
    d. 250

91. The Consumer-Patient Radiation Health and Safety Act functions in each of the following *except* _____.
    a. mandating the number of radiographic exposures for specific treatment
    b. establishing guidelines for the proper maintenance of x-ray equipment
    c. requiring persons who take dental radiographs to be properly trained and certified
    d. outlining requirements for the safe use of dental x-ray equipment

92. With size 2 film, a total of _____ anterior film placements are used with the paralleling technique.
    a. four
    b. six
    c. seven
    d. eight

93. Which size film is traditionally used with the bisecting technique?
    a. No. 1 film for anterior teeth, No. 1 film for posterior teeth
    b. No. 1 film for anterior teeth, No. 2 film for posterior teeth
    c. No. 2 film for anterior teeth, No. 1 film for posterior teeth
    d. No. 2 film for anterior teeth and for posterior teeth

94. When vertical posterior bitewing exposures are indicated, size _____ film is placed with the long portion of the film in a _____ direction.
    a. 1, horizontal
    b. 2, horizontal
    c. 1, vertical
    d. 2, vertical

95. Which of the following choices may be the cause of an unexposed film?
    a. excessive exposure time
    b. failure to turn on the x-ray machine
    c. excessive kilovoltage
    d. excessive milliamperage

96. When the occlusal technique is used, _____ to stabilize the film.
    a. a Stabe Bite-Block is used
    b. a hemostat is used
    c. the patient gently bites on the surface of the film
    d. a bitewing tab is used

97. When using the occlusal technique, the film is positioned with the _____ side facing the arch that is being exposed, and the film is placed in the mouth _____.
   a. white, to the lingual of the teeth
   b. white, between the occlusal surfaces of the maxillary and mandibular teeth
   c. colored, to the lingual of the teeth
   d. colored, between the occlusal surfaces of the maxillary and mandibular teeth

98. In panoramic radiography, the _____ rotates around the patient.
   a. film
   b. tubehead
   c. tubehead and film
   d. dental chair

99. To help reduce the gag reflex:
   a. tell the patient to hold his or her breath
   b. try to reduce tactile stimuli
   c. use the term "gagging" when talking with the patient
   d. do not try to distract the patient

100. _____ digital imaging involves digitizing an existing x-ray film using a CCD camera. Indirect digital imaging is _____ to direct digital imaging.
   a. Indirect, inferior
   b. Direct, inferior
   c. Indirect superior
   d. Direct, superior

Infection Control

Directions: Select the response that best answers each of the following questions. Only one response is correct.

1. Which of the following is a special type of microorganism that is highly resistant to heat and chemicals?
   a. yeasts
   b. viruses
   c. spores
   d. staphylococci

2. Which of the following microorganisms is the smallest?
   a. cocci
   b. viruses
   c. yeasts
   d. bacilli

3. What does the term "CFU" mean?
   a. counts found undetermined
   b. colony-forming units
   c. coli forming units
   d. counts first undertaken

4. What mode of disease transmission is a needle stick?
   a. direct contact
   b. indirect contact
   c. droplet infection
   d. airborne infection

5. In a dental office, what is most efficient transmission mode of hepatitis B virus?
   a. direct transmission
   b. indirect transmission
   c. droplet infection
   d. airborne infection

6. The most important source of infectious microorganisms in a dental office is:
   a. practitioner's hands
   b. airborne particles
   c. water
   d. patients' mouths

7. What are standard precautions?
   a. considering all patients to have infections with a bloodborne pathogen
   b. use of the same infection control procedures for all types of health care facilities
   c. considering that blood and all patient body fluids are potentially infectious
   d. using only infection control procedures formally approved by a government agency

8. An emerging disease is one that:
   a. is caused by an unknown virus
   b. almost always occurs in children
   c. was not previously recognized
   d. is fatal in almost all cases

9. Which of the following is not a mode for spread of HIV/AIDS?
   a. sexual contact
   b. mother to newborn
   c. percutaneous
   d. inhalation

10. What is the risk of occupational acquisition of HIV/AIDS by dental assistants?
   a. very high
   b. high
   c. modest
   d. very low

11. Which of the following is *not* a bloodborne pathogen?
   a. hepatitis A virus
   b. hepatitis B virus
   c. hepatitis C virus
   d. HIV

12. Which of the following has the longest incubation time?
   a. hepatitis A virus
   b. hepatitis B virus
   c. hepatitis C virus
   d. HIV

13. Which of the following is most likely to cause infection after an exposure?
   a. hepatitis A virus
   b. hepatitis B virus
   c. hepatitis C virus
   d. HIV

14. The best protection against a hepatitis B infection is:
   a. engineering control
   b. vaccination
   c. work practice control
   d. wearing gloves

15. Herpetic whitlow is an infection of the:
   a. oral cavity
   b. hands/fingers
   c. eyes
   d. genitals

16. Tuberculosis spreads best by:
   a. inhalation
   b. ingestion
   c. mucous membrane contact
   d. breaks in the skin

17. Which government agency requires employers to protect their employees from exposure to patient blood and other body fluids?
   a. Environmental Protection Agency
   b. Centers for Disease Control and Prevention
   c. Food and Drug Administration
   d. Occupational Safety and Health Administration

18. Which government agency regulates the effectiveness of sterilizers?
   a. Environmental Protection Agency
   b. Centers for Disease Control and Prevention
   c. Food and Drug Administration
   d. Occupational Safety and Health Administration

19. Which government agency regulates surface disinfectants?
   a. Environmental Protection Agency
   b. Centers for Disease Control and Prevention
   c. Food and Drug Administration
   d. Occupational Safety and Health Administration

20. Can you return teeth to patients without disinfection?
   a. yes
   b. no

21. Which of the following is dedicated to infection control in dentistry?
   a. Association for Advancement of Medical Instrumentation
   b. American Dental Assistants Association
   c. Organization for Safety and Asepsis Procedures
   d. Association of Professionals in Infection Control and Epidemiology

22. How often should you receive the influenza vaccine?
   a. once
   b. twice a year
   c. once a year
   d. every 10 years

23. From the list below, select the best procedure for caring for a handpiece.
   a. steam under pressure with emulsion
   b. steam under pressure without emulsion
   c. cold chemical/immersion

24. How often should you receive the tetanus vaccine?
   a. once a year
   b. every 2 years
   c. every 5 years
   d. every 10 years

25. Paying the costs of vaccinating at-risk employees against hepatitis B is the responsibility of:
   a. the employee
   b. the employer
   c. insurance company
   d. the federal government

26. For which of the following is there currently no available vaccine?
   a. hepatitis B
   b. hepatitis C
   c. influenza
   d. mumps

27. What is the last piece of personal protective equipment put on before treating a patient?
   a. mask
   b. clinical gown
   c. protective eyewear
   d. gloves

28. What is the first piece of personal protective equipment taken off after treating a patient?
   a. mask
   b. clinical gown
   c. protective eyewear
   d. gloves

29. What type of gloves should you wear when assisting during the placement of an amalgam?
   a. sterile surgical
   b. utility
   c. examination
   d. nonmedical

30. What is the most common skin reaction to the wearing of gloves?
   a. irritant contact dermatitis
   b. allergic contact dermatitis
   c. latex hypersensitivity

31. Surgical masks used in dentistry:
   a. protect against exposure to TB
   b. totally prevent the inhalation of dental aerosols
   c. prevent spatter from contacting mucous membranes
   d. are required only when treating adults

32. Bacterial filtration efficiency is a measure of effectiveness for:
   a. gloves
   b. masks
   c. protective eyewear
   d. protective clothing

33. When do you need to change your protective clothing?
    a. after every patient
    b. each half-day of work
    c. when visibly soiled
    d. after using a high-speed handpiece

34. Removal of which of the following is required when temporarily leaving the operatory?
    a. protective clothing
    b. protective eyewear
    c. surgical mask
    d. gloves

35. From the list below, select the best procedure for caring for a contaminated needle.
    a. steam under pressure with emulsion
    b. steam under pressure without emulsion
    c. sharps container
    d. discard in biohazard container

36. When is it appropriate to use an alcohol-based hand rub?
    a. only if a sink is available
    b. only if used before another handwashing agent
    c. only if used after another handwashing agent
    d. only when there is no visible soil on the hands

37. How long should you rub your hands when washing with soap and water?
    a. around 3 minutes
    b. no more than 5 seconds
    c. at least 15 seconds
    d. exactly 45 seconds

38. From the list below, select the best procedure for caring for a tube of cavity liner.
    a. steam under pressure with emulsion
    b. steam under pressure without emulsion
    c. discard
    d. spray/wipe/spray with surface disinfectant

39. Which of the following should be worn while cleaning contaminated instruments?
    a. heavy-duty utility gloves and protective clothing
    b. a mask, heavy-duty utility gloves, and protective eyewear and clothing
    c. a mask, examination gloves, and protective eyewear and clothing
    d. protective eyewear, a mask, and heavy-duty utility gloves

40. What is the leading cause of sterilization failure in dental offices?
    a. mechanical malfunction
    b. poorly constructed instruments
    c. human error
    d. selection of wrong type of sterilizer

41. What is the reason for holding (presoaking) instruments prior to cleaning?
   a. kill microorganisms
   b. reduce water spotting
   c. make cleaning easier
   d. minimize rusting

42. What is the reason for cleaning instruments prior to sterilization?
   a. increase chances of sterilizer success
   b. reduce instrument rusting and dulling
   c. kill any microorganisms present
   d. minimize instrument damage

43. When using an ultrasonic cleaner, which of the following is a *correct* procedure?
   a. Routine cleaning takes about 60 seconds.
   b. Use a basket for loose instruments or a basket or rack for cassettes.
   c. Hand scrub instruments before placement in the ultrasonic cleaner.
   d. Use dishwashing detergents, they work and are cheaper.

44. What is the rationale for packaging instruments prior to sterilization?
   a. helps minimize instrument rusting and dulling
   b. reduces instrument damage from occurring
   c. maintains instrument sterility after processing
   d. helps in organizing instruments into functional groups

45. Which of the following combinations will produce the greatest amount of instrument rusting and dulling?
   a. carbon steel instruments in a steam sterilizer
   b. stainless steel instruments in an unsaturated chemical vapor sterilizer
   c. carbon steel in a dry heat sterilizer
   d. stainless steel instruments in a steam sterilizer

46. Which sterilizer is best biologically monitored by *Bacillus atrophaeus* (*subtilus*) spores?
   a. dry heat sterilizers
   b. steam autoclaves
   c. unsaturated chemical vapor sterilizers

47. Which of the following has the highest operating temperature and longest cycle time?
   a. dry heat sterilizers
   b. steam autoclaves
   c. unsaturated chemical vapor sterilizers

48. According to the CDC, how often should you biologically monitor your sterilizer?
   a. each load
   b. weekly
   c. monthly
   d. every 2 months

49. Recording the highest temperature reached during a sterilization cycle is an example of _____ monitoring.
   a. physical/mechanical
   b. chemical
   c. biological

50. How often should you use chemical monitors in your sterilizer?
   a. with every instrument pack
   b. with one pack per load
   c. daily
   d. weekly

51. Which is the following is *not* acceptable for use as a surface disinfectant in a dental office?
   a. iodophors
   b. chlorine-based products
   c. glutaraldehydes
   d. phenolics

52. Which of the following best describes an intermediate-level surface disinfectant?
   a. sporicidal agent
   b. bacteriocidal agent
   c. virucidal agent
   d. tuberculocidal agent

53. What should you do before disinfecting a clinical contact surface?
   a. wipe the surface with a high-level disinfectant
   b. clean the surface
   c. cover with plastic for at least 10 minutes
   d. nothing; just go ahead and disinfect

54. Which of the following terms indicates the highest level of killing power?
   a. sporicidal agent
   b. bacteriocidal agent
   c. virucidal agent
   d. tuberculocidal agent

55. Which of the following is *not* a clinical contact surface?
   a. unit light handle
   b. bracket table switch
   c. sink in the treatment room
   d. air/water syringe

56. What would you do to a clinical contact surface after removal of a plastic surface cover before the next patient?
   a. Clean and disinfect with an intermediate-level disinfectant and place a new cover.
   b. Clean and disinfect with a low-level disinfectant and then add a new cover.
   c. Clean and disinfect with a high-level disinfectant and recover.
   d. If no contamination is present, then place a new plastic cover.

57. How often should you replace the plastic cover placed over the light handles?
   a. after every patient
   b. at least every half-work day
   c. when the cover becomes visibly soiled
   d. only when damage to cover has occurred

58. Which of the following can kill bacterial spores, tuberculosis, and viruses?
   a. low-level disinfectants
   b. intermediate-level disinfectants
   c. high-level disinfectants

59. You should *not* use which of the following as a cover barrier for a bracket table?
   a. aluminum foil
   b. paper sheet
   c. plastic sheet
   d. plastic bag

60. Which of the following is the major disadvantage of using bleach as a surface disinfectant?
   a. cannot kill HIV
   b. expensive
   c. not effective against TB
   d. adverse reactions with metals

61. Which of the following best describes the Spaulding Classification System?
   a. ranks resistance of microorganisms to chemical disinfectants
   b. ranks instruments as to their potential to cause infection
   c. ranks disinfectants as to their ability to kill tuberculosis
   d. ranks the reaction by healthcare workers to disinfectants

62. What is the maximum acceptable level of bacteria in dental unit water as recommended by the CDC?
   a. 700 CFU/ml
   b. 900 CFU/ml
   c. 500 CFU/ml
   d. 400 CFU/ml

63. Which of the following best defines the term *potable water?*
   a. sterile water
   b. dental unit water
   c. drinking water
   d. chlorinated water

64. How often does the CDC recommend flushing of dental unit water lines?
   a. between every patient
   b. at the beginning of the workday
   c. at the beginning and end of the workday
   d. at least three times a day

65. What should you do before changing or cleaning a vacuum line trap?
   a. Do nothing.
   b. Remove and then heat sterilize the vacuum line.
   c. Flush bleach through the line and follow with a water flush.
   d. Evacuate a disinfectant-detergent into the line and flush with water.

66. Patient-to-patient cross-contamination may occur when a patient closes his or her lips around which of the following?
  a. air/water syringe tip
  b. saliva ejector tip
  c. high-volume evacuator tip
  d. metal prophy angle

67. Which of the following is a disadvantage of using disposable items?
  a. It does not always prevent patient-to-patient transfer of microorganisms.
  b. There is no need to process hard to sterilize items.
  c. Performance may be less efficient than their reusable counterparts.
  d. It may be more expensive than reusable types.

68. Patient care instruments are categorized into various classifications. Into which classification would instruments such as blood pressure cuffs, pulse oximeter, and stethoscope be placed?
  a. critical
  b. semicritical
  c. noncritical

69. Ideally, when should you disinfect an impression?
  a. chairside
  b. in the office lab
  c. upon arrival at the dental lab
  d. just before leaving the dental lab

70. You should not use which of the following to disinfect a full denture prior to sending it off to the dental lab?
  a. iodophors
  b. diluted bleach
  c. quaternary ammonium compounds
  d. phenolics

71. Air suction motors on dental lathes should produce an air velocity of at least:
  a. 50 ft/min
  b. 200 ft/min
  c. 650 ft/min
  d. 1500 ft/min

72. What should you do if your x-ray positioners cannot be autoclaved?
  a. Throw them away and get some that can be autoclaved.
  b. Enclose them using a plastic wrapping material.
  c. Soak them in a high-level disinfectant.
  d. Clean them carefully with soap and water.

73. What should you do when using a daylight loader?
  a. Keep some disinfect inside the loader to treat film packets.
  b. Only open the film packets after they are in the loader.
  c. Only open film packets inside of plastic pouches inside the loader.
  d. Insert only disinfected or unsoiled film packets.

74. Which of the following is an example of regulated medical waste?
   a. used examination gloves
   b. disposable clinic gowns
   c. used anesthetic needles
   d. used masks

75. A sharps container is an example of a(n):
   a. administrative control
   b. work practice control
   c. engineering control
   d. personal protective equipment

76. Which of the following is *not* a recognized type of regulated medical waste?
   a. extract teeth
   b. sharps
   c. used PPE
   d. liquid blood

77. Regulated medical waste comprises what percentage of a dental office's total waste?
   a. 1% to 2%
   b. around 5%
   c. 20% to 25%
   d. 40%

78. What should you do if the outside of a biohazard bag becomes contaminated?
   a. Process it through a steam autoclave.
   b. Disinfect the outside surface.
   c. Place it into the regular trash.
   d. Place it inside another biohazard bag.

79. How would you properly sterilize filled sharps containers in-house?
   a. Process teeth with and without amalgam.
   b. Use the usual cycle tine.
   c. Process containers on their sides.
   d. Process containers with their vents open.

80. What federal agency requires employers to inform employees of their risk and to offer free the hepatitis B vaccine?
   a. Centers for Disease Control and Prevention
   b. Occupational Safety and Health Administration
   c. Food and Drug Administration
   d. Environmental Protection Agency

81. According to OSHA, which of the following is most effective in protecting employees while at work?
   a. administrative controls
   b. engineering controls
   c. personal protective equipment
   d. work practice controls

82. Which of the following is a specific eye, mouth, other mucous membrane, nonintact skin, or parenteral contact with blood or other potentially infectious materials that results from the performance of an employee's duties?
    a. needle stick accident
    b. nosocomial infection
    c. exposure incident
    d. contamination

83. After initial training, how often must employees receive training concerning the OSHA Bloodborne Pathogens Standard?
    a. monthly
    b. twice a year
    c. at least annually
    d. only if needed

84. According the Spaulding Classification System, dental explorers are:
    a. critical instruments
    b. semicritical instruments
    c. noncritical instruments

85. Why is it important to dry instrument packages inside the sterilizer after the end of a sterilization cycle?
    a. prevents wicking of microbes through wet packaging
    b. prevents instruments from sticking to each other
    c. prevents water spots from forming on instruments
    d. allows chemical indicators to work properly

86. How would you minimize corrosion of carbon steel instruments during sterilization?
    a. Use a steam autoclave or a dry heat sterilizer.
    b. Use an unsaturated chemical vapor sterilizer or a steam autoclave.
    c. Place in a liquid sterilant such as glutaraldehyde.
    d. Use a dry heat sterilizer or an unsaturated chemical vapor sterilizer.

87. What is the purpose of the Hazard Communication Standard?
    a. provide patients with information concerning their care
    b. inform employees of their chemical risks at work
    c. provide the public with chemical safety information
    d. help manufacturers improve their MSDS

88. Who provides MSDS?
    a. employer
    b. office employees
    c. OSHA
    d. chemical's manufacturer

89. How many sections are there in an MSDS?
    a. 6
    b. 7
    c. 8
    d. 9

90. What must you have for every hazardous chemical in your work environment?
    a. a matching MSDS
    b. a specific warning sign
    c. the amount present in the workplace
    d. flammability designation

91. There is a diamond-shaped symbol on the bottle of a chemical in your office. Its red-colored section
    has the number four written inside. What does this mean?
    a. The chemical poses a modest health hazard to workers.
    b. The chemical is normally unstable and can undergo rapid violent change.
    c. The chemical is more expensive that other similar types.
    d. The chemical vaporizes quickly at room temperature and burns readily.

92. According to the Hazard Communication Standard, employees must receive training at the time of
    their initial assignment and then:
    a. at least weekly
    b. upon introduction of a new hazard
    c. every month
    d. every other year

93. You should *not* consider which of the following to be a hazardous chemical?
    a. bleach
    b. ethyl alcohol
    c. aspirin
    d. amalgam

94. Who designates a chemical as being hazardous?
    a. employers
    b. the EPA
    c. employees
    d. manufacturers

95. A hospital level disinfectant is the same as a(n):
    a. high-level disinfectant
    b. intermediate-level disinfectant
    c. low-level disinfectant

96. What is the goal of infection control?
    a. reduce the number of microorganisms shared between people
    b. increase the human body's resistance to microorganisms
    c. decrease the virulence of all microorganisms
    d. sterilize all instruments used on patients

97. Which of the following procedures helps protect both a dental assistant and dental patients?
    a. wearing protective eyewear
    b. wearing gloves
    c. wearing a protective gown
    d. proper surface disinfection

98. You must remove which of the following when temporarily leaving a seated patient?
   a. surgical mask
   b. protective eyewear
   c. gloves
   d. protective clothing

99. Which of the following is the least desirable method for cleaning dental instruments?
   a. instrument washer
   b. hand scrubbing
   c. ultrasonic cleaner

100. Use of liquid sterilants, such as glutaraldehyde, is restricted to what type of reusable items?
   a. metal
   b. blood contaminated
   c. heat sensitive
   d. critical level

Answer Keys and Rationales

TEST 3

General Chairside

1. In the universal lettering system for primary teeth, which letter stands for the maxillary left second molar?
   b. The letter J stands for the maxillary left second molar in the universal lettering system for primary teeth. K stands for the mandibular left second molar; T stands for the mandibular right second molar; and C stands for the maxillary right canine.

2. The type of caries that occurs on the occlusal surfaces or the buccal and lingual grooves of posterior teeth is(are) _____.
   c. Pit and fissure caries can occur on occlusal surfaces, buccal and lingual grooves of posterior teeth, or the lingual pits of the maxillary incisors. Smooth surface caries occurs on intact enamel other than pits and fissures; root surface caries occur on any surface of the root; secondary caries, also known as recurrent caries, occur on the tooth surrounding a restoration.

3. Which of the following is *not* one of the components of the ABCDs of basic life support?
   a. The ABCDs of basic life support stand for airway, breathing, circulation, and defibrillation.

4. What does this charting symbol indicate?
   a. A gold crown is indicated by outlining the crown of the tooth and placing diagonal lines in it.

5. Which surgical procedure describes a hemisection?
   d. A hemisection is a procedure in which the root and crown are cut lengthwise and removed. Removal of the apical portion of the root is an apicoectomy; the removal of diseased tissue through scraping is apical curettage; the removal of one or more roots without removing the crown is a root amputation.

6. What does this charting symbol indicate?
   b. A missing tooth is indicated by drawing an X through the tooth.

7. What does this charting symbol indicate?
   d. Veneers only cover the facial aspect of a tooth and are indicated by outlining the facial portion only.

8. The respiration rate for an adult who has just participated in an aerobic activity might be:
   d. A person who has just completed an aerobic activity such as water aerobics or running would have an increased pulse that could range from 80 to 110.

9. What does this charting symbol indicate?
   b. A fracture is indicated with a red zigzag line.

10. Using Black's classification of cavities, a lesion on the cervical third of a tooth is considered a class _____ restoration or cavity.
    d. A Class V carious lesion or restoration is found at the cervical third of the tooth.

11. The abbreviation used in the progress notes or chart to indicate a mesioocclusodistal restoration with a buccal extension would be:
   c. Each surface is given an initial and in the naming of this restoration the surfaces are in the sequence of mesial, occlusal, distal, and buccal—thus, MODB.

12. When working with anesthetic needles, the _____ the gauge number, the thicker is the needle.
   b. The gauge refers to the thickness of the needle. The smaller the gauge number, the thicker is the needle. A large gauge number indicates a thinner needle.

13. The hard palate is recorded in the _____ impression.
   b. The hard palate and tuberosities are reproduced in the maxillary impression. The retromolar area is reproduced in the mandibular impression.

14. The tooth-numbering system that uses a two digit tooth recording system with the first digit indicating the quadrant and the second digit indicating the tooth within the quadrant, with numbering from the midline to the posterior is referred to as the:
   c. The Fédération Dentaire Internationale System is the only system that uses two digits in the number with the first digit indicating the quadrant and the second digit indicating the tooth within the quadrant, with numbering from the midline to the posterior.

15. Which of the following statements is *not* true as it relates to a patient's respiration?
   d. Respirations are normally lower in count per minute than the pulse rate. For instance the normal pulse rate is between 60 and 80 and the respirations per minute is between 14 and 18.

16. The respiration pattern of a patient in a state of tachypnea has:
   b. The respiration pattern of a patient in a state of tachypnea is excessively short, rapid breathes.

17. The respirations of a patient who is hyperventilating will be exemplified by:
   c. When a patient is hyperventilating, the respirations will be abnormally fast and deep.

18. A patient who displays symptoms of unconsciousness, increased body temperature, rapid heart beat, and increased blood pressure may be displaying symptoms of:
   b. Common symptoms of a grand mal seizure include unconsciousness, increased body temperature, rapid heartbeat, and increased blood pressure. These symptoms may be preceded by an aura or by localized spasm or twitching of muscles.

19. If a patient displays symptoms of hypoglycemia and is conscious, what is the first thing you should ask the patient?
   b. You must determine when the patient last ate and if insulin has been taken before proceeding with any treatment.

20. The MyPyramid is an outline of what to eat each day. The smallest segment of the pyramid is:
   d. The smallest segment of the pyramid is composed of oils.

21. Any food that contains sugars or other carbohydrates that can be metabolized by bacteria in plaque is described as being:
   b. Cariogenic foods are those that contain sugars or other carbohydrates that can be metabolized by bacteria in plaque to cause dental decay.

22. Organic substances that occur in plant and animal tissues are _____, and essential elements that are needed in small amounts to maintain health and function are _____.
   c. Vitamins are organic substances that occur in plant and animal tissues, and minerals are essential elements that are needed in small amounts to maintain health and function. Both are essential for good health and body function.

23. A horizontal or transverse plane divides the body into:
    a. When a body is divided horizontally, it will produce an upper and a lower portion or superior and inferior portions.

24. Which of these instruments is a combination DE instrument used as an explorer and periodontal probe?
    d. An expro is a double-ended instrument designed to be used as an explorer on one end and a periodontal probe on the opposite end.

25. The forceps are used in this portion of the clamp while placing the rubber dam.
    b. The tips of the rubber dam forceps are placed in the holes to grasp the clamp and expand it to fit over the tooth during rubber dam placement.

26. Which of the following statements is *false* as it relates to correct use of the HVE tip?
    c. HVE tips are available in metal and plastic materials, with some being sterilizable and others being disposable.

27. The water-to-powder ratio generally used for an adult maxillary impression is _____ measures of water, _____ scoops of powder.
    a. The water-to-powder ratio used for an adult maxillary impression is generally three measures of water and three scoops of powder.

28. High velocity evacuation provides all *except* which of the following?
    a. High-volume evacuation does not increase the patient's desire to rinse as it removes fluids rapidly from the patient's mouth.

29. Which of the following statements is *not* a concept of four handed dentistry?
    d. Wide-winged dental chairs prohibit the operator and assistant from getting close to the patient, thus causing undue back and neck strain.

30. The _____ handpiece can operate both forward and backward and can be used with a variety of attachments.
    c. The low-speed handpiece can operate both forward and backward and is able to hold a variety of angles and contra-angles for slow cutting, polishing, and abrading.

31. When the Tofflemire matrix band retainer is used which of the knobs or devices would be used to adjust the size or loop of the matrix band to fit around the tooth and loosen the band for removal?
    d. The inner knob, D, adjusts the size or the loop of the matrix band to fit around the tooth and loosens the band for removal.

32. Which of the following instruments is a K style file?
    b. The K type root canal file in B is used to clean and contour the inside walls of the root canal.

33. Which of the following instruments would be used to remove debris or granulation tissue from a surgical site?
    b. The surgical curette is designed with spoonlike working ends that enable it to be used to easily remove debris and granulation tissue from the surgical site.

34. Which of he following statements is *true* when using a Tofflemire matrix band and retainer?
    b. For ease of use, the operator places the matrix retainer on the buccal surface of the prepared tooth, and the wedge is placed from the lingual at the proximal surface involved.

35. The dental team is completing an amalgam procedure on 4^{MOD}. Which of the following statements is *true*?
    b. Two proximal walls are involved; thus, two wedges will be needed to secure the matrix band. Anatomical carvers will be used because the occlusal surface is involved.

36. When a two paste system is used for a composite material, the paste of either jar should not be cross contaminated because:
   a. By placing the contents of one jar into the other jar a chemical reaction will occur causing the material to harden.

37. Which of the following statements is *false* true as it relates to the acid etching of enamel for a composite restoration?
   b. According to manufacturer's directions the acid-etching agent is not rubbed vigorously on the surface.

38. When cleaning a dental handpiece, it is important to:
   a. Failure to follow the manufacturer's directions while cleaning a handpiece can render the handpiece ineffective and may alter the warranty.

39. Which of the following rotary instruments would cut faster and most efficiently?
   c. A diamond stone is designed to provide maximum cutting capabilities. The diamond flecks on the tip of the instrument are one of the hardest materials available for bur design.

40. Which classification of motions should the dentist and the dental assistant eliminate to increase productivity and decrease stress and body fatigue?
   d. Class IV and V motions require the greatest amount of movement at chairside and should be eliminated in order to reduce stress and increase productivity.

41. Which of the following conditions is *not* a potential medical contraindication to nitrous oxide?
   d. All of the answers in a through c impact the use of nitrous oxide. Age is not a contraindication of the use of this substance.

42. What substance is added to a local anesthetic agent to slow down the intake of the agent and increase the duration of action?
   b. A vasoconstrictor is used to slow down the intake of the anesthetic agent and increase the duration of the action of the local anesthesia.

43. The type of anesthesia achieved by injecting the anesthetic solution directly into the tissue at the site of the dental procedure is known as _____.
   c. Infiltration anesthesia is achieved by injecting the anesthetic solution directly into the tissue at the site of the dental procedure and is generally used on the maxillary teeth because of the porous nature of the alveolar cancellous bone.

44. General anesthesia is most safely administered in a(an):
   c. General anesthesia is most safely administered in a hospital setting or another facility with the necessary equipment for administration and the management of an emergency.

45. An orthodontic positioner is designed to:
   b. An orthodontic positioner is a custom appliance that fits over the patient's dentition after orthodontic treatment to retain the teeth in their desired position and permit the alveolus to rebuild support around the teeth before the patient wears a retainer.

46. Which of these would *not* be a choice of instrument to place gingival retraction cord?
   a. The explorer has sharp pointed beaks that would not be conducive to the placement of gingival retraction cord.

47. From the photo below, identify the procedure for which this tray would be used?
   b. This tray is assembled to assist in the delivery and cementation of a cast restoration. The bite stick, articulating paper, and Backhaus towel forceps all are clues to this set up.

48. The instruments shown below from left to right are:
   b. The photographs shown from left to right are the Howe pliers, wire bending pliers, and ligature tying pliers. There are no bird beak pliers, posterior band remover, or ligature cutters shown.

49. To control bleeding after a surgical procedure, the patient should be instructed to do all of the following *except* _____.
  d. Rinsing will cause bleeding to be accelerated and may cause a clot to become lose. Pressure should be used for at least 30 minutes, and strenuous work and physical activity restricted for a day.

50. What is the endodontic test in which the dentist applies pressure to the mucosa above the apex of the root and notes any sensitivity or swelling?
  b. The palpation test is performed by applying pressure to the mucosa above the apex of the root and noting any sensitivity or swelling. The percussion test is performed by tapping on the tooth in question; thermal sensitivity, or the cold test, is performed by isolating the tooth in question and applying a source of cold to determine a response. Electric pulp testers test a tooth's vitality with a small electric stimulus.

51. The process by which the living jawbone naturally grows around the implanted dental supports is known as:
  c. An osseointegration is used to attach living healthy bone to a dental implant.

52. The treatment used as an attempt to save the pulp and encourage the formation of dentin at the site of the injury is a(n):
  a. Pulp capping is the process of applying a dental material to a cavity preparation with an exposed or nearly exposed dental pulp in an attempt to encourage the formation of dentin at the injury site.

53. The removal of the coronal portion of an exposed vital pulp is a(n):
  b. A pulpotomy is the removal of the coronal portion of a vital pulp from a tooth. This is a procedure indicated for vital primary teeth, teeth with deep carious lesions, and emergency situations.

54 The instrument used to adapt and condense gutta-percha points into the canal during endodontic treatment is:
  b. The spreader or plugger is used in the canal to compact the gutta-percha points as they are placed.

55. The surgical removal of diseased gingival tissues is called:
  b. The gingivectomy is the surgical removal of diseased gingival tissues, whereas the gingivoplasty is a surgical reshaping and contouring of these tissues.

56. A(n) _____ is a dentist with a license in the specialty of dentistry that provides restoration and replacement of natural teeth and supporting structures.
  d. A prosthodontist is a dentist with a license in the ADA recognized specialty of dentistry that provides restoration and replacement of natural teeth and supporting structures.

57. Periodontal pocket depth is charted at _____ points on each tooth during a baseline charting procedure.
  c. Six points on the tooth are charted for periodontal depth in determining a baseline: mesiobuccal, buccal, distobuccal, distolingual, lingual, and mesiolingual.

58. A periodontal pocket marker is similar in design to a _____.
  b. The periodontal pocket marker appears like cotton pliers but has beaks at right angles to enable marking to take place on the gingival tissue.

59. A(n) _____ is an additive bone surgery that includes the reshaping and contouring of the bone.
  b. An osteoplasty is a surgical procedure in which bone is added, contoured, and reshaped.

60. From the instruments shown below, select the periosteal elevator.
  a. The periosteal elevator is a double-ended instrument with flat and sharp ends that enable the dentist to loosen the gingival tissue and to compress the alveolar bone surrounding the neck of the tooth.

61. Using Black's classification of cavities, a pit and fissure lesion on the occlusal surface of molars and premolars is considered a class _____ cavity.
  a. Class I lesions or restorations are found in the pit and fissure areas on the occlusal surface of molars and premolars.

62. Using Black's classification of cavities, a pit lesion on the buccal surface of molars and premolars is considered a class _____ restoration or cavity.
    a. Class I lesions or restorations are found in the pit and fissure areas on the buccal and lingual surfaces of molars and premolars as well as on the occlusal surfaces of these teeth.

63. The more fixed attachment of the muscle that is usually the end attached to the more rigid part of the skeleton is the:
    a. The origin of a muscle is the end attached to the more rigid part of the skeleton, whereas the insertion of the muscle is the movable attachment of the distal end of the muscle.

64. Which of the following teeth would *not* be found in the deciduous dentition?
    c. There are no premolars present in the primary dentition.

65. A redline is used on this tooth. What does this charting symbol indicate?
    b. Red diagonal lines through a tooth indicate it is to be extracted.

66. What does this charting symbol indicate?
    a. Recurrent decay is indicated by outlining an existing restoration.

67. On a cephalometric analysis, the abbreviation Na stands for:
    c. The abbreviation Na stands for nasion on a cephalometric analysis.

68. Which orthodontic pliers are used in fitting bands for fixed or removable appliances?
    b. Contouring pliers are used for fitting bands for fixed or removable appliances. Bird beak pliers are used in forming and bending wires; posterior band remover pliers remove bands without placing stress on the tooth; Howe pliers are used in placement and removal or creation of adjustment bends in the arch wire.

69. If the charting conditions indicate that there is a furcation involvement some type of symbol will be placed at the:
    c. A furcation is the area between two or three roots. Thus, if a tooth has a furcation involvement, a horizontal line is drawn at this site.

70. A reproduction of an individual tooth on which a wax pattern may be constructed for a cast crown is a(n):
    a. The reproduction of an individual tooth is called a "die." Upon this single model, a wax pattern is constructed to make the image for the cast crown.

71. Which of the following materials would *not* be used to take a final impression for the creation of a prosthetic device?
    c. Alginate hydrocolloid is not a material of choice for a final impression for which some form of prosthetic device is to be made. This impression material may be used for study models but does not have the strength or accuracy of the other listed materials.

72. A porcelain fused to metal crown would be designed so the porcelain would always be on the _____ surface.
    b. The porcelain would appear on the buccal/facial surface of a tooth that is to be covered with porcelain fused to metal for aesthetic reasons.

73. A glass ionomer material may be used for all of the following *except* a(n):
    d. Glass ionomer material does not have an obtundant or soothing characteristic.

74. If the room temperature and humidity are very low while mixing a final impression material the setting time may be:
    b. A cool dry environment will allow more working time when mixing a dental impression material; thus, the setting time is increased.

75. A porcelain fused to metal crown is being seated. The assistant will mix the cement to a _____ or _____ consistency.
    d. When seating a porcelain fused to metal crown, the cement to be mixed must be of a thin consistency, referred to as a cementation consistency. This consistency is also referred to as the primary consistency rather than secondary, which is a thicker firmer material.

76. A posterior tooth with a deep preparation may require a base that is designed to prepare pulpal defense by functioning is a(n):
    c. To protect the pulp, the dental cement provides insulation to the tooth from temperature and other environmental factors.

77. A patient has a fractured amalgam on 29DO. Time in the doctor's schedule does not permit placement of a permanent restoration. Which of the following statements is *correct* as to the type of dental cement and the consistency that would be used in this clinical situation?
    a. Because a permanent restoration will be placed at a later date, a temporary restoration will be placed at this appointment. The patient will be biting on this restoration during normal mastication, and thus it must be a firm heavy material as in a secondary consistency.

78. An alginate impression has been taken to prepare a set of diagnostic models. Which of the following statements is *false* as it relates to handling the impression? Alginate impressions_ _____.
    d. Alginate impressions may not be stored in 100% relative humidity as the impression will absorb the moisture fairly quickly and the physical dimension of the impression will change. This type of impression should be stored in a moist towel for only a short period of time.

79. IRM (Intermediate restorative material) is used primarily for:
    b. A provisional restoration is a temporary restoration, and the IRM material functions only as a temporary restoration for a period of time before a permanent restoration can be placed on the tooth.

80. Dry mouth is also known as _____.
    c. Xerostomia is known as dry mouth caused by the reduction of saliva.

81. _____ is more prominent in older adults who have experienced gingival recession.
    b. Cervical caries is of concern for elderly persons, who often have gingival recession. Carious lesions on root surfaces form more quickly than do coronal caries because cementum on the root surface is softer than enamel or dentin.

82. Which food can be compared to a reversible hydrocolloid?
    c. Ice cream is a reversible hydrocolloid. A change in temperature causes the material to transform from one physical state to another. When the ice cream is frozen, it is in the gel state. When left at room temperature, the ice cream melts and turns into a sol state. When reurned to the freezer, the ice cream again becomes a gel.

83. Which of the following could *not* be suggested as an intervention for the prevention of dental caries?
    d. Chewing mints, although saliva could be stimulated, is not a suggestion intervention for prevention of dental caries. Mints contain sugar and this adds to the potential increase in dental caries.

84. A caries risk assessment test is used to determine the number of_____.
    a. A caries risk assessment test is used to determine the mutans streptococci and lactobacilli count in the saliva.

85. Inflammation of the supporting tissues of the teeth that begins with _____ can progress into the connective tissue and alveolar bone that supports the teeth and become _____.
    c. A patient may develop gingivitis in the oral cavity and without intervention of improved oral hygiene, necessary dental care, and changes in diet, this condition can progress into periodontitis.

86. A dietary food analysis includes a diary of everything a patient consumes for:
    a. A dietary analysis is completed by a patient for everything they consume within 24 hours. Some dentists may ask to have this completed over several days, but the 24-hour base is used as the basic format.

87. The MyPyramid is an outline of what to eat each day. Which of the following statements is *true* regarding a food pyramid:
    c. Recent research has provided a food pyramid for a vegetarian diet that provides similar suggestions in the pyramid format for those patients who are vegetarians.

88. From the photograph below, which of these instruments is a T-ball burnisher?
    a. The T-ball burnisher has a flat end on one side of the instrument with a ball on the other side. It is used to burnish margins after placing an amalgam restoration.

89. The patient's record indicates that the status of the gingiva is bulbous, flattened, punched-out, and cratered. This statement describes the gingival _____:
    b. *Bulbous, flattened, punched-out,* and *cratered* are all terms that are used to describe gingival contour.

90. Supragingival calculus is found on the _____ of the teeth, above the margin of the _____.
    b. Supragingival calculus is found on the clinical crowns above the margin of the gingiva. The prefix *supra* means "above."

91. Subgingival calculus occurs _____ the gingival margin and can be _____ in color due to subgingival bleeding
    d. Subgingival calculus occurs below the gingival margin; *sub* refers to "below" or "beneath." The color is black due to the subgingival bleeding.

92. All of the following are types of restorations *except* _____.
    b. The classes of restorations are Class I, II, III, IV, and V.

93. _____ sealants _____ require mixing as they cure when they are exposed to UV light.
    d. Light cured sealants do not require mixing as they cure when they are exposed to UV light, unlike chemically cured sealants, which require mixing in order for the material to cure.

94. When adjusting a crown after cementation, the dentist most likely would use a(n) _____.
    c. A stone is commonly used to adjust the crown after cementation as it will gently reduce the surface that needs to be adjusted without damaging the restoration.

95. The procedure that is done to remove subgingival calculus and to remove necrotic tissue from the periodontal pocket is referred to as a(n) _____:
    d. A gingival curettage is the procedure that involves scraping or cleaning the gingival lining of the pocket with a sharp curette to remove necrotic tissue from the pocket wall.

96. The _____ provides rapid calculus removal and reduces operator hand fatigue.
    c. The ultrasonic scaler is a mechanical device that provides rapid vibrations to remove calculus and reduce the operator hand fatigue.

97. A(n) _____ procedure is performed to remove defects and to restore normal contours in the bone.
    c. Osseous surgery is the procedure performed to remove defects and to restore normal contours to the bone. The other procedures all relate to soft tissue surgery.

98. Which of the following is *not* a measurement used in constructing a complete denture?
    d. Reversion is not a term used in dentistry in relation to denture construction.

99. When transferring patient records from the office to another site, the administrative assistant must do all *except* which of the following?

    c. Patient records are not sent in their entirety to another site. These records must remain in the office. Only information that is requested and for which consent is given may be transferred.

100. A new filing system for clinical charts is to be installed in your office. Which of the following filing systems would be most efficient?

    a. Open files with colored filing labels using alpha and numeric codes are the most common and efficient method for paper records storage. The other systems require more time and motion to use.

101. If an administrative assistant chooses to transmit a transaction about a patient electronically, under which act does this task fall?

    c. The Health Insurance Portability and Accountability Act (HIPAA) of 1996 specifies federal regulations ensuring privacy regarding a patient's health care information.

102. A message about a serious illness or allergy should be noted in which manner on the clinical record?

    b. To protect a patient's privacy, information about a serious illness or allergy must be placed inside the record in a discreet but obvious manner such as a small brightly colored label.

103. The group responsible for establishing regulations that govern the practice of dentistry within a state is the:

    d. The Board of Dentistry in each state is responsible for establishing regulations that govern the practice of dentistry within each state. The membership and appointment of the members of these boards may vary from state to state.

104. The act of doing something that a reasonably prudent person would not do or not doing something that a reasonably prudent person would do is:

    c. Negligence is the performance of an act that a reasonably careful person under similar circumstances would not do or conversely, the failure to perform an act that a reasonable careful person would do under similar circumstances.

105. The universal retainer is also referred to as the _____ retainer.

    a. The universal retainer is also referred to as the Tofflemire retainer. It is a device that holds the matrix band snugly in position.

106. A clinical dental assistant is hired in the practice. The dentist indicates that this person is to place an intracoronal provisional restoration. The person knows how to perform the task but does not yet have the EFDA credential required to perform the specific intraoral task. What should you suggest to her when she asks you what she should do?

    c. A clinical dental assistant should perform only those tasks that are legally assigned by state law and for which they are appropriately educated. If requested to do otherwise, it is the assistant's responsibility to inform the dentist that they are not legally qualified to perform a specific task.

107. The Good Samaritan Law offers incentives for healthcare providers to provide medical assistance to injured persons without the fear of potential litigation except under which of the following circumstances?

    a. The Good Samaritan law was considered necessary to create an incentive for health care providers to provide medical assistance to the injured in cases of automobile accidents or other disasters without the fear of potential litigation. The law is intended for individuals who do not seek compensation but rather are solely interested in providing care to the injured in a caring, safe manner, with no intent to do bodily harm.

108. The objectives of good appointment book management include all *except* which of the following?

    d. A good appointment book management system provides maximum productivity, reduction of staff tension, a concern for patient needs, and minimum downtime.

109. In reference to appointment management, prime time refers to:

    b. Prime time is the most requested time. This may vary from community to community. Most commonly, it is time after school or after work.

110. Which time of day is considered most appropriate when treating young children?

    c. Early morning time is a good time to schedule a young child as they are more alert and refreshed. Trying to schedule a child during playtime or naptime can be strenuous for the caregiver.

111. What type of supply is a curing light used in a dental office?

    b. A curing light is a nonexpendable item because it can be reused and is not very expensive, like a capital item of several thousands of dollars.

112. A patient has the following amalgam restorations: 29MO, 30^{MOD}, 31DO, and 32°. The fee for each surface is $115. What is the fee for services rendered?

    d. The per surface fee is multiplied by 8 surfaces, and the total fee for service is $920.

113. Light curing:

    b. Light curing is used to polymerize composite resin materials and composite resin cement. It relies on visible light since ultraviolet light was proven to be damaging to the operator's eyes. Light curing is not used to polymerize silver dental amalgam. Self-cured composites are auto-polymerized. Auto-polymerized composite resin materials require mixing prior to placement.

114. The tip of the composite curing light should be held at an angle of __ degrees to the tooth.

    a. The tip of the composite curing light should be held at an angle of 90 degrees to the tooth. The depth of cure is affected by the angle of the light.

115. Composite restorative materials are usually cured for __ seconds with the halogen curing light.

    b. Composite restorative materials are usually cured for 20 seconds with the halogen curing light. Some newer, high intensity lights cure composite restorative material in less time. Composite core material is usually cured for 60 seconds. It is always important to follow the manufacturer's recommendations regarding curing time.

116. The removable denture prosthesis can be cleaned in the dental office by all of the methods listed below EXCEPT:

    d. Any one of the first three techniques may be used to clean a removable denture prosthesis in the dental office. Immersion in an ultrasonic cleaner with a special denture solution is an excellent way to remove plaque and debris. Brushing with a denture brush is also effective for accessible areas. Some patients will form tenacious calculus on dentures and this can be removed by the dental hygienist with hand scalers and curettes. It would not be an effective method to attempt to clean the denture prosthesis in the patient's mouth.

117. A broken removable denture prosthesis can be repaired:

    c. A broken removable denture prosthesis can be repaired in the office with cold-cured acrylics. The patient should be discouraged from home repair since there is often only one chance to correctly approximate the relationship between the broken pieces. Once the patient has "melted" the acrylic and placed the denture pieces in an incorrect relationship it is usually impossible to repair the denture properly and a new denture must be fabricated.

118. _____ cement must be mixed on a glass slab.

    c. Zinc phosphate cement must be mixed on a glass slab. Zinc polycarboxylate cement may be mixed on a glass slab or paper.

Zinc oxide-eugenol cement can be mixed on a glass slab or on oil resistant paper. Calcium hydroxide cement can be mixed on a glass slab or on paper.

119. Which of the following materials is recommended for polishing filled hybrid composites and resin restorations?

    b. Aluminum oxide paste is recommended for polishing filled hybrid composites and resin restorations.

120. A maxillary denture _____ have a full palate and a mandibular denture _____ have a full palate.

    b. A maxillary denture will have a full palate and a mandibular denture will not have a full palate.

Radiation Health and Safety

1. The_____ film provides a view that shows the bony and soft tissue areas of the facial profile.

    d. The cephalometric radiograph provides a view of the bones of the face and skull as well as the soft tissue profile of the face and is used by the orthodontist in diagnosis.

2. In digital radiography, the sensor replaces the _____.

    c. In digital radiography, the sensor is a small detector that is placed intraorally to capture a radiographic image, thus replacing intraoral dental film.

3. Digital radiography requires _____ x-radiation than conventional radiography because the sensor is _____ sensitive to x-rays than conventional film.

    a. Digital radiography requires less x-radiation than conventional radiography. Less x-radiation is necessary to form a digital image on the sensor because the typical sensor is more sensitive to x-rays than conventional film.

4. Examples of conditions resulting in smooth root resorption are _____ and _____.

    b. Examples of conditions resulting in smooth root resorption are tumors and cysts.

5. Who is the guardian of a patient's dental records?

    c. The dentist is the guardian and keeper of dental records, and the records are property of the dentist. Patients may request a copy of their radiographs from the dentist.

6. The _____ radiograph is the film of choice for the intraoral examination of large areas of the upper or lower jaw.

    a. A radiographic occlusal examination is used to inspect large areas of the maxilla or mandible on one film.

7. The _____ radiograph is the film of choice for the extraoral examination of the upper or lower jaw.

    d. The panoramic film is an extraoral radiograph that is designed to provide a wide view of the maxilla and mandible on a single film.

8. A(n) _____ is a lesion characterized by a localized mass of granulation tissue around the apex of a nonvital tooth; appears radiolucent.

   b. The periapical granuloma appears radiolucent or dark on a radiograph and is characterized by a localized mass of granulation tissue around the apex of a nonvital tooth.

9. The most common cause of poor definition in a radiograph is _____,

   c. Movement influences film sharpness. A loss of image sharpness occurs if either the film or the patient moves during the x-ray exposure.

10. A film that has been fogged will have decreased:

   a. A fogged film will have decreased contrast.

11. Presently, the maximum permissible dose (MPD) for dental workers with ionizing radiation is _____.

   b. Radiation protection standards dictate the maximum dose of radiation that an individual can receive. The maximum permissible dose (MPD) for occupationally exposed persons who work with radiation is 5.0 rem/year.

12. Light leaks in a darkroom will cause:

   c. Fogged films result from improper safe lighting and light leaks in the darkroom as well as improper film storage, outdated films, contaminated processing solutions, and high developer temperature.

13. The types of radiation interaction with patients include all of the following *except* _____.

   c. Tertiary is not a type of radiation interaction that would apply to patient exposure.

14. If the radiographic processing time is too short, the film will appear _____.

   b. If a film is underdeveloped, it will appear light. To prevent underdeveloped films, be certain to check the temperature as well as the time the film remains in the developer solution.

15. Which is the correct sequence for processing x-ray film?

   b. The sequence of the steps in processing a film that has been exposed includes development, rinsing, fixing, rinsing, and drying.

16. The developing agent in the developer solution is:

   a. The developing agent (also known as the reducing agent) contains two chemicals: hydroquinone (paradihydroxybenzene) and elon (monomethylpara–aminophenol sulfate)

17. An overdeveloped film may be caused by which of the following?

   c. When a film is overdeveloped, it has had excessive development time and will appear dark. To avoid this condition, check the temperature of the developer and decrease the time the film remains in the developer as needed.

18. When using the bisecting techniques, the imaginary angle that is bisected is formed between the long axis of the tooth and the:

   c. The bisecting technique is based on a simple geometric principle known as the rule of isometry. This geometric principle is applied to the bisecting technique used in dental radiography to form two imaginary equal triangles. The bisecting technique requires that the following be accomplished: the film must be placed along the lingual surface of the tooth; at the point where the film contacts the tooth, the plane of the film and the long axis of the tooth form an angle; the radiographer visualizes a plane that divides in half, or bisects, the angle formed by the film and the long axis of the tooth; and the central ray of the x-ray beam is directed perpendicular to the imaginary bisector.

19. An application of tomography used in dentistry is:

   c. TMJ tomography provides the most definitive imaging of the TMJ's bony components. As a result, the condyle, articular eminence, and glenoid fossa can all be examined on a tomogram. This image can also be used to estimate joint space and evaluate the extent of movement of the condyle when the mouth is open.

20. _____ enables viewing of an area in three planes
    b. Computed tomography allows for the imaging of one layer or section of the body while blurring images from structures in other planes.

21. What would a fluoride artifact look like on a radiograph?
    b. Some fluorides, especially stannous fluoride, will produce black marks on radiographs.

22. On intraoral radiographs, when the patient's right is on your left, the identification dot on the film will be:
    a. When the raised side of the identification dot is facing the viewer, the radiographs are then being viewed from the labial aspect. The patient's left side is on the viewer's right and the patient's right side is on the viewer's left side as if the viewer is looking directly at the patient.

23. A completed root canal would appear _____ _____ on processed radiographs.
    a. A completed root canal will appear radiopaque whether the filling is done with gutta-percha or silver points. The gutta-percha appears less radiodense than the silver point.

24. Which of the following will appear radiopaque on a radiograph?
    d. A cement base will appear radiopaque. Compared to a metal restoration, however, the cement base will be less radiodense.

25. A supernumerary tooth in the midline is referred to as a(n):
    b. A supernumerary tooth, often paired, that has a small cone-shaped crown and a short root and appears between the maxillary central incisors is referred to as a mesiodens.

26. Which of the following statements is *not* true about a bitewing radiograph?
    c. The central ray of the x-ray beam is directed through the contacts of the teeth, using a vertical angulation of 110 degrees.

27. If a lead apron is folded after being used, it will _____ and _____.
    b. Lead aprons and thyroid collars must not be folded when stored. Folding eventually cracks the lead and allows radiation leakage.

28. The lead apron is:
    a. The lead apron is a flexible shield placed over the patient's chest and lap to protect the reproductive and blood-forming tissues from scatter radiation; the lead prevents the radiation from reaching these radiosensitive organs. It is recommended for intraoral and extraoral film exposures and is mandated in many states.

29. Added filtration in the dental x-ray tubehead:
    d. Added filtration refers to the placement of aluminum disks in the path of the x-ray beam between the collimator and the tubehead seal in the dental x-ray machine. Filtration of the x-ray beam results in higher energy and more penetrating useful beam.

30. _____ is used to restrict the size and shape of the x-ray beam and to reduce patient exposure.
    c. Collimation is used to restrict the size and shape of the x-ray beam and to reduce patient exposure. A collimator, or lead plate with a hole in the middle, is fitted directly over the opening of the machine housing where the x-ray beam exits the tubehead.

31. The radiopaque restoration on the first molar is:
    b. An amalgam restorations on the mandibular first molar that has an overhang at the mesial cervical region.

32. What is the landmark indicated by the arrows?
    c. The internal oblique ridge appears as a radiopaque band that extends downward and forward from the ramus.

33. What is evident in this film?
    b. Physiologic resorption is shown in this film. This is a process that is seen with the normal shedding of primary teeth.

34. What is evident in this panoramic film?
    c. The panoramic film in this question illustrates the metal framework for both maxillary and mandibular partial dentures with porcelain teeth in the posterior quadrants of both arches.

35. When the voltage is increased:
    c. When voltage is increased, the speed of the electrons is increased. When the speed of the electrons is increased and the electrons strike the target with greater force and energy, resulting in a penetrating x-ray beam with a short wavelength.

36. What is the landmark indicated by the arrows?
    a. The coronoid process appears as a triangle-shaped opacity. It is a marked prominence of bone on the anterior ramus of the mandible. It does not appear on a mandibular periapical radiograph but does appear on the maxillary molar periapical film.

37. In which two lengths are PIDs typically available?
    c. Position-indicating devices or cones appear as an extension of the x-ray tubehead and are used to direct the x-ray beam. They are typically available in two lengths: short (8 inches) and long (16 inches).

38. When a pregnant patient expresses concern about the need for radiographs, which of the following statements should be used?
    d. The response in d recognizes the patient's concern and lets her know that there is concern for the fetus and that only the x-rays that are essential for immediate treatment are to be taken.

39. Which processing error results in the "herringbone effect"?
    c. Film reversal results in the herringbone effect, a light film with a geometric pattern from the lead foil embossed on it.

40. What is the restoration on the mandibular first molar?
    b. Stainless steel crowns are prefabricated restorations that are usually used as a temporary restoration. These crowns are thin and will not absorb dental x-rays to the extent that an amalgam or a cast restoration would. Thus, the stainless steel crown appears radiopaque but not as dense as amalgam or gold.

41. What is the restoration on the maxillary lateral incisor?
    c. All porcelain crowns appear slightly radiopaque on a dental radiograph. A thin radiopaque line outlining the prepared tooth may be evident through the slightly radiopaque porcelain crown. The thin line represents cement used to seat the crown.

42. What is the restoration on the maxillary arch?
    b. A porcelain fused to metal bridge has two radiographic components: the metal component and a porcelain component. The metal appears completely radiopaque, and the porcelain component appears slightly radiopaque.

43. The "unsharpness," or blurring, that surrounds the edges of a radiographic image is the _____ _____.
    b. Penumbra is from the Latin *pene*, meaning "almost," and *umbra*, meaning "shadow". In relation to a radiograph, it refers to the unsharpness, or blurring of the edges of a radiographic image.

44. _____ radiation is the penetrating x-ray beam that is produced at the target of the anode.
    c. Primary radiation refers to the penetrating x-ray beam that is produced at the target of the anode and then exits the tubehead. Other terms for primary radiation are *primary beam* and *useful beam*.

45. _____ radiation is that form of radiation that is in the environment and includes cosmic and terrestrial radiation.
    d. Background radiation comes from natural sources such as radioactive materials in the ground and cosmic radiation from space.

46. The median palatine suture appears _____ in a radiograph.
  a. On a maxillary periapical radiograph, the median palatine suture appears as a thin radiolucent line between the maxillary incisors.

47. The film mounting method in which radiographs are placed in the film mouth with the depressed side of the identification dot facing the viewer is referred to as _____ mounting.
  a. This system of film mounting is not used frequently, but when it is used, the dental professional then views the radiographs from the lingual aspect, as if the viewer were sitting on the inside of the patient's mouth and looking out; the patient's left side is on the viewer's left side and the patient's right side is on the viewer's right side.

48. The lead tubular device used to restrict the size and shape of the x-ray beam is the lead _____.
  c. The collimator is a diaphragm, usually lead, that is used to restrict the size and shape of the x-ray beam.

49. The _____ is a unit of measurement for dose equivalent; the SI unit equivalent to the rem.
  b. Sievert (Sv) is the unit of measurement for dose equivalent; the SI unit of measurement equivalent to the rem; 1 Sv5100 rem.

50. Regressive alteration of tooth structure that occurs within the crown or root of a tooth and appears radiolucent in a radiograph is _____ _____.
  b. Internal resorption occurs within the crown or root of the tooth and involves the pulp chamber, pulp canals, and surrounding dentin. This type of resorption is often caused by trauma, pulp capping, and pulp polyps.

51. Which of these would *not* be a maxillary landmark for the maxilla in a panoramic view?
  d. The mental foramen is an opening or hole in the bone located on the external surface of the mandible in the region of the premolars. It would appear as a small ovoid or round radiolucent area located in the apical region of the mandibular premolars.

52. Extraoral radiography will be used for all of the following *except* to _____.
  c. Extraoral radiography is not the film of choice for diagnosing dental caries. Bitewing radiographs are used for this procedure.

53. If the _____ is not placed on the _____ ___during a panoramic radiographic exposure, a radiolucent shadow will be superimposed over the apices of the maxillary teeth.
  b. It is necessary for the patient to raise the tongue to the roof of the mouth during panoramic exposure to avoid a radiolucent shadow being superimposed over the apices of the maxillary teeth.

54. A _____ lead apron is recommended for use during the exposure of a panoramic film.
  b. A double-sided lead apron is used for panoramic exposures in order to protect the front and the back of the patient. A thyroid collar is not used as it blocks part of the beam and can obscure important diagnostic information.

55. _____ film is used in panoramic radiography.
  a. Screen film is used in panoramic radiograph. This type of film is sensitive to the light that is emitted from the intensifying screens.

56. Size 3 film is _____ and is used only for _____ images.
  b. Size 3 film is longer and narrower than the standard size 2 film and is used only for bitewing images.

57. The sizes available for bitewing film include:
  b. Film sizes for bitewing radiography range from 0 to 3 and vary according to use, dentist preference, and the size of the patient.

58. Size 0 film is most commonly used on:
  a. Size 0 film is used primarily for children as it is only $\frac{7}{8} \times \frac{13}{8}$ inches in size.

59. The image shown in this projection is a:
  b. This is a mandibular pediatric occlusal project. The incomplete closure of the apical region and the mixed dentition aid in this determination.

60. The image shown in this projection would require the patient be positioned with the mandibular arch:
    a. The patient is positioned with the mandibular arch parallel to the floor for this exposure and the central ray is directed at −55 degrees to the plane of the film.

61. Which type of dentition best describes this radiograph?
    c. A child would be in a mixed dentition status when the teeth of both dentitions are present.

62. When exposing a molar bitewing, the following conditions should exist *except* _____.
    c. The anterior edge of the film should be placed at the midline of the mandibular second premolar to ensure that all the molars will be present in the molar bitewing film.

63. The image shown above the teeth in this projection is a(n):
    b. Nose jewelry appears on this film as a radiopacity and corresponds in size and shape of the object that is being worn by the patient.

64. A severe carious lesion on a x-ray will:
    c. A severe carious lesion on a radiograph will extend through the enamel and dentin and more than half the distance toward the pulp. This may also be classified as a Class IV lesion.

65. Root caries involves:
    b. Root caries does not involve the enamel; it involves the cementum and dentin only.

66. An anterior periapical film is oriented _____, and a posterior periapical film is oriented _____.
    a. To ensure that all the apical regions and the entire tooth are visible on a periapical film, the film is place vertically for an anterior periapical film and horizontally for a posterior periapical film.

67. Which of the following is an advantage of digital radiography?
    c. One of the greatest advantages of digital radiography is for the dentist to be able to view the radiograph more quickly.

68. A concept of radiation protection that states that all exposure to radiation must be kept to a minimum is _____.
    a. ALARA is a concept of radiation protection that states that all exposure to radiation must be kept to a minimum or "as low as reasonably achievable."

69. The _____ governs the orientation of structures portrayed in two radiographs exposed at different angulations.
    b. The buccal object rule governs the orientation of structures portrayed in two radiographs exposed at different angulations. The buccal object rule can be used to determine the position of a root canal when there are multiple canals or to identify the position of a canal filled with gutta-percha in a maxillary tooth with two or more roots.

70. The arrows indicate the _____ in this image.
    b. The median palatine suture appears as a thin radiolucent line in this film.

71. What is the error in this film?
    a. A cone cut is seen when the PID is not properly aligned with the bitewing film-holding device.

72. What is the error in exposure of this film?
    b. The images are distorted in this film, and this was caused by incorrect vertical angulation.

73. What is the error in exposure of this film?
    c. The film shows incorrect film placement for the molar bitewing.

74. Which of the following definitions is *incorrect?*
    c. A right angle is formed by two lines perpendicular to each other or an angle at 90 degrees.

75. What do you respond when the patient asks who owns the dental radiographs?

c. The dentist owns the x-rays, but the patient may request a copy of these radiographs or a copy can be sent to a dentist of the patient's choice.

76. A fogged film appears:

a. A fogged film appears gray and lacks image detail and contrast. This condition can result from improper safe lighting and light leaks in a darkroom, improper film storage, outdated films, or even contaminated processing solutions.

77. Static electricity appears as _____ on a film.

d. A film with thin, black branching lines has been subjected to static. This is caused by opening a film packet too quickly or opening a film packet before touching another object, such as a countertop in a carpeted office. This condition occurs more commonly during low humidity times.

78. Which of the following statements is *not* correct concerning the exposure sequence for periapical films?

b. The dental radiographer should always have an established exposure routine to prevent errors and use the time most efficiently. Failure to do this may result in omitting an area or exposing it twice. Routinely, when using the paralleling technique for periapical films, always start with the anterior teeth first on the maxillary and then on the mandible. When working from the right to the left in the maxillary arch and then left to right in the mandibular arch, no wasted movement or shifting of the PID occurs. After anterior films are exposed, the premolar and molar films can be exposed, again using an efficient system of placement.

79. What piece of equipment is required to hold the film parallel to the long axis of the tooth in the paralleling technique?

b. When using the paralleling technique, it is necessary to use some type of film holder. A variety of film holders are available, some designed for one-time use and others that are sterilizable.

80. What size film is used with the posterior XCP instrument?

c. Commonly, size 1 film is used in the anterior and size 2 is used in the posterior regions.

81. What is the error in exposure of this film?

a. The error in this film is foreshortening, as the teeth appear short with blunted roots. To avoid this error, do not use excessive vertical angulation with the bisecting technique. The use of a Rinn instrument minimizes such errors in the paralleling technique.

82. What person is responsible for the final and definitive interpretation of dental radiographs?

a. Only the dentist is responsible for the final diagnosis of the radiographs and the interpretation for the patient. The assistant and hygienist must be skilled in recognition of the various pathologic conditions, anatomic landmarks, and common errors and may identify these for a patient but are not licensed to make a final interpretation and diagnose.

83. An explanation of what is viewed on a radiograph is _____, whereas the identification of a disease by examination and analysis is _____.

b. Diagnosis and interpretation have very different meanings and should not be interchanged. To *interpret* is to explain what is viewed on a radiograph, and to *diagnose* is to identify a disease by examination and analysis. In dentistry, the diagnosis is made by the dentist after a thorough review of the medical history, dental history, clinical examination, radiographic examination, and any clinical or laboratory tests performed.

84. The nucleus of an atom contains:

c. The nucleus of the atom, or dense core of the atom, is composed of particles known as protons and neutrons. Protons carry positive electrical charges and neutrons carry no electrical charge.

85. Which of the following statements is *true* regarding the direct theory of radiation injury?

  c. The direct theory of radiation injury is defined as the cell damage that results when ionizing radiation directly hits critical areas within a cell. Therefore, if the x-ray photons directly strike the DNA of a cell, critical damage can occur, resulting in injury to the irradiated organism.

86. _____ regulate(s) the manufacture and installation of dental x-ray equipment.

  d. All x-ray machines must meet specific federal guidelines regulating diagnostic equipment performance standards. The state and local governments may regulate how dental x-ray equipment is used and dictate codes that pertain to the use of x-radiation. Dependent on the local and state safety codes, dental equipment must be inspected and monitored routinely.

87. Which of the following statements is *true* regarding the placement of a film packet in the patient's mouth?

  a. The tube side of the film is white and has a raised bump in one corner and, when placed in the mouth, the white side faces the teeth and the tubehead. The label side of the film packet has a flap and is color coded to identify films outside of the plastic packaging container; when placed in the mouth, the color-coded side of the packet must face the tongue.

88. During formation of the latent image, irregularities in the lattice structure of the exposed crystal, known as the _____, attract silver atoms.

  c. During latent image formation, some silver bromide crystals and exposed and energized, while other crystals are not exposed. The irregularity in the lattice structure of the exposed crystal is known as sensitivity specks and attracts silver atoms.

89. Radiographs are a(n) _____ comprehensive patient care.

  a. Radiographs are a vital component to comprehensive patient care. The old adage, "To see is to know, not to see is to guess," applies to this concept.

90. With faster F-speed film, a single intraoral film results in a surface skin exposure of _____ milliroentgens.

  c. With the development of F speed film, the surface exposure, or the measure of the intensity of radiation on a patient's skin surface, has decreased significantly. Today, a single intraoral radiograph results in a mean surface exposure of 100 mR compared to the exposure of D-speed film a few years ago of 250 mR.

91. The Consumer-Patient Radiation Health and Safety Act functions in each of the following *except* _____.

  a. The Consumer Patient Radiation Health and Safety Act is designed to establish guidelines for the use and maintenance of x-ray equipment, not to dictate the number or type of radiographs to be taken for each patient. This latter duty is the responsibility of the dentist.

92. With size 2 film, a total of _____ anterior film placements are used with the paralleling technique.

  b. With size 2 film, six films will be used for anterior exposures: three on the maxillary and three on the mandible.

93. Which size film is traditionally used with the bisecting technique?

  d. Size 2 film is used in both the anterior and posterior regions when using the bisecting technique. In the anterior, the film is placed in a vertical direction, and in the posterior, in a horizontal direction.

94. When vertical posterior bitewing exposures are indicated, size _____ film is placed with the long portion of the film in a _____ direction.
    d. Size 2 film may be used for all exposures. The film is bitewing and is placed with the long portion of the film in a vertical direction.

95. Which of the following choices may be the cause of an unexposed film?
    b. An unexposed film will appear clear and can be caused by failure to turn on the x-ray machine, electrical failure, or malfunction of the x-ray machine.

96. When the occlusal technique is used, a _____ to stabilize the film.
    c. When the occlusal technique is used, the patient need only gently bite on the film; no other devices are necessary.

97. When using the occlusal technique, the film is positioned with the _____ side facing the arch that is being exposed, and the film is placed in the mouth _____.
    b. To expose an occlusal film, the film is placed between the occlusal surfaces of both arches with the white side facing the arch that is being exposed.

98. In panoramic radiography, the _____ rotates around the patient.
    c. When a panoramic radiograph is exposed, the tubehead and film rotate around the patient, while the patient remains stable.

99. To help reduce the gag reflex:
    b. To prevent the patient from gagging, it is necessary to avoid any tactile stimuli to the gag reflex area.

100. _____ digital imaging involves digitizing an existing x-ray film using a CCD camera. Indirect digital imaging is _____ to direct digital imaging.
    a. Indirect digital imaging is the method of obtaining a digital image in which an existing radiograph is scanned and converted into a digital form using a CCD camera. This method does not provide the same quality as would direct imaging.

Infection Control

1. Which of the following is a special type of microorganism that is highly resistant to heat and chemicals?
    c. There are some bacteria that have developed a defense mechanism against death caused by adverse environmental conditions. A spore is a dense thick-walled structure that enables the cell to withstand unfavorable environmental conditions. The spore or endospore is one of the most resistant forms of life against heat, drying, and chemicals.

2. Which of the following microorganisms is the smallest?
    b. Viruses are smaller than bacteria, ranging from 0.02 μm to 0.3 μm. Bacteria can range from 0.2 μm up to 1 μm wide and 5 to 10 mm up to 30 μm long.

3. What does the term "CFU" mean?
    b. The term CFU refers to colony-forming units, or small groups of cells.

4. What mode of disease transmission is a needle stick?
    b. Indirect transmission of disease results from injuries with contaminated sharps, such as needle sticks, or other contaminated instruments.

5. In a dental office, what is most efficient transmission mode of hepatitis B virus?
    b. The most efficient means of transmitting hepatitis B in the dental office is via indirect contact with items contaminated with the patient's microorganisms such as surfaces, hands, and contaminated sharps.

6. The most important source of infectious microorganisms in a dental office is:

   d. The major source of disease agents in the dental office is from the mouths of the patients. Microorganisms can be a source of contamination in other areas of the office, but by far the patient's mouth presents the greatest source.

7. What are standard precautions?

   c. Standard precautions means to consider blood, all body fluids including secretions and excretions (except sweat), nonintact skin, and mucous membranes as potentially infectious in all patients.

8. An emerging disease is one that:

   c. Emerging diseases are new infectious diseases that until this time have not been recognized or are known infectious diseases with changing patterns.

9. Which of the following is not a mode for spread of HIV/AIDS?

   d. HIV/AIDS is transmitted by intimate sexual contact, exposure to blood, blood contaminated body fluids, or blood products, and perinatal contact.

10. What is the risk of occupational acquisition of HIV/AIDS by dental assistants?

   d. Studies of occupation risks of HIV infection for health care workers indicate the risk of occupational acquisition of HIV/AIDS is very low for this category of workers.

11. Which of the following is *not* a bloodborne pathogen?

   a. Hepatitis A does not pose an occupational risk for dental workers or patients because this form of hepatitis is spread primarily by the fecal-oral route involving consumption of contaminated food or water.

12. Which of the following has the longest incubation time?

   d. The incubation time for HIV is the longest of the viruses listed, sometimes lasting for several months or even years.

13. Which of the following is most likely to cause infection after an exposure?

   b. The evolution of the protective vaccine for hepatitis B is attributed to the decrease in the number of HBV infections found in dental health care workers. The unvaccinated members of the dental team are at least 2 to 5 times more likely to become infected with HBV than the general population.

14. The best protection against a hepatitis B infection is:

   b. Studies have shown a significant decrease in HBV infections when the dental health care worker is vaccinated against this disease.

15. Herpetic whitlow is an infection of the:

   b. Herpetic whitlow is an infection of the fingers with herpes simplex virus. It is uncommon today because dental health care workers routinely wear gloves during treatment.

16. Tuberculosis spreads best by:

   a. The primary route of transmission is inhalation. Spread from one person to another relates to the closeness of contact and the duration of the exposure to infectious droplets.

17. Which government agency requires employers to protect their employees from exposure to patient blood and other body fluids?

   d. The Occupational Safety and Health Administration's (OSHA) bloodborne pathogens standard is the most important infection control law in dentistry for the protection of the health care workers.

18. Which government agency regulates the effectiveness of sterilizers?

   c. The purpose of the FDA is to ensure the safety and effectiveness of drugs and medical devices by requiring "good manufacturing practices" and reviewing the devices against associated labeling to ensure that claims can be supported.

19. Which government agency regulates surface disinfectants?
    a. The EPA is associated with infection control by attempting to ensure the safety and effectiveness of disinfectants. Information on the safety and effectiveness of disinfectants must be submitted by manufacturers to the for review to make sure that safety and antimicrobial claims stated for the products are supported by scientific evidence.

20. Can you return teeth to patients without disinfection?
    a. Extracted teeth should be disposed of as regulated medical waste unless they are returned to the patient.

21. Which of the following is dedicated to infection control in dentistry?
    c. OSAP, founded in 1984 and formally incorporated as a nonprofit organization in 1986, is considered the resource for dentistry for infection control and occupational safety and health.

22. How often should you receive the influenza vaccine?
    c. For their own well-being and the health of their patients and families, the dental health care worker should receive the influenza vaccine annually.

23. From the list below, select the best procedure for caring for a handpiece.
    b. To ensure sterilization of this device, it should be placed in steam under pressure without the use of emulsion. Always be certain that the selected sterilization method meets the recommendations of the dental manufacturer.

24. How often should you receive the tetanus vaccine?
    d. The CDC Advisory Committee on Immunization Practices recommends that boosters need to be given only every 10 years.

25. Paying the costs of vaccinating at-risk employees against hepatitis B is the responsibility of:
    b. In accord with the OSHA Bloodborne Pathogens Standard, hepatitis B vaccination performance standards states that the employer must provide information on the vaccine, including the efficacy, safety, and method of administration, as well as the benefits of being vaccinated and the assurance that all medical records concerning the vaccination process will be kept confidential. In addition, the vaccine is to be provided by the employer and be given under the supervision of a physician.

26. For which of the following is there currently no available vaccine?
    b. Vaccines do not exist for all diseases from which the dental health care worker is exposed. Hepatitis C is one of the diseases for which there is currently no vaccine available.

27. What is the last piece of personal protective equipment put on before treating a patient?
    d. Gloves are the last piece of personal protective equipment that should be put on before treating a patient.

28. What is the first piece of personal protective equipment taken off after treating a patient?
    b. When removing personal barriers, the disposable gown would be removed first, and it is pulled off over gloved hands, turning it inside out and immediately placing it into a waste receptacle. Avoid touching any underlying clothes when removing protective clothing.

29. What type of gloves should you wear when assisting during the placement of an amalgam?
    c. During routine patient care, the dental health are worker wears disposable latex or nonlatex examination gloves.

30. What is the most common skin reaction to the wearing of gloves?

   a. Most reactions from wearing gloves result from nonimmunologic irritation of the skin from nonlatex chemicals in the gloves or applied to the hands. When irritant contact dermatitis occurs the skin on the hands becomes dry, reddened, itchy, and sometimes cracked.

31. Surgical masks used in dentistry:

   c. In dentistry, the masks primarily protect the mucous membranes of the nose and mouth from aerosol sprays and spatter of oral fluids from the patient or from items contaminated with patient fluids.

32. Bacterial filtration efficiency is a measure of effectiveness for:

   b. Face masks are composed of synthetic material that aids in filtering out at least 95% of small particles that directly contact the mask.

33. When do you need to change your protective clothing?

   c. Microorganisms from aerosols, sprays, splashes, and droplets from the oral fluids of patients not only contaminate eyes and mucous membranes of the nose and mouth but also contaminate other body sites, including the forearms and chest area. Outer protective clothing can protect against this contamination. When the outer clothing is obviously contaminated, it should be changed before providing care for another patient.

34. Removal of which of the following is required when temporarily leaving the operatory?

   d. If the dental health care worker leaves the chairside during treatment, the gloves must be removed and a fresh pair placed prior to returning to chairside. An alternative is to place a pair of overgloves before leaving the chair and removing these before returning.

35. From the list below, select the best procedure for caring for a contaminated needle.

   c. A contaminated needle is placed in the sharps container.

36. When is it appropriate to use an alcohol-based hand rub?

   d. When hands contain no visible soil, alcohol-based hand rubs without water and without rinsing have been shown to be effective in hand antisepsis.

37. How long should you rub your hands when washing with soap and water?

   c. Scrub hands, nails, and forearms using a liquid antimicrobial handwashing agent and soft brush for at least 15 seconds.

38. From the list below, select the best procedure for caring for a tube of cavity liner.

   d. Medicaments such as cavity liners can be disinfected by spray/wipe/spray or using a disinfectant wipe and wiping first to clean and a second time to disinfect.

39. Which of the following should be worn while cleaning contaminated instruments?

   b. Utility gloves, protective eyewear, mask, and protective clothing are all worn during instrument processing. These barriers will provide personal protection from contaminants on the instruments and from the chemicals being used.

40. What is the leading cause of sterilization failure in dental offices?

   c. The primary cause of sterilization failure is human error; improper loading, improper timing, improper cleaning, improper packaging, or selecting the wrong sterilization method are all caused by human error.

41. What is the reason for holding (presoaking) instruments prior to cleaning?

   c. Precleaning reduces the bioburden on the instrument, and this may insulate microorganisms from the sterilizing agent. A dirty instrument will not become sterile.

42. What is the reason for cleaning instruments prior to sterilization?

   a. Cleaning instruments prior to sterilization will ensure proper sterilization. The FDA has approved ultrasonic cleaners and instrument washers for this purpose.

43. When using an ultrasonic cleaner, which of the following is a *correct* procedure?
    b. Manufacturers of ultrasonic cleaners recommend using a basket for loose instruments or a basket or rack for cassettes.

44. What is the rationale for packaging instruments prior to sterilization?
    c. By wrapping or packaging instruments prior to sterilization, the risk of poststerilization contamination is reduced.

45. Which of the following combinations will produce the greatest amount of instrument rusting and dulling?
    a. Carbon steel instruments placed in steam sterilization will promote rusting and dulling. This can be prevented by using distilled water in the sterilizer and a protective emulsion.

46. Which sterilizer is best biologically monitored by *Bacillus atrophaeus* (*subtilus*) spores?
    a. To monitor a dry heat sterilizer, it is recommend that *Bacillus atrophaeus* strips be used.

47. Which of the following has the highest operating temperature and longest cycle time?
    a. The dry heat sterilizer requires 60 to 120 minutes of processing at a temperature of 320° F.

48. According to the CDC, how often should you biologically monitor your sterilizer?
    b. The CDC, ADA, and OSAP, as well as the Association for the Advancement of Medical Instrumentation, recommend at least weekly spore testing of each sterilizer in the office. Some states require routine spore testing of dental office sterilizers.

49. Recording the highest temperature reached during a sterilization cycle is an example of _____ monitoring.
    a. The personal monitoring/observation and recording of sterilizer activity are considered physical/mechanical monitoring.

50. How often should you use chemical monitors in your sterilizer?
    a. Appropriate monitoring as recommended by the CDC involves the use of a chemical indicator on the inside and outside (if the internal indicator cannot be seen) of each pack, pouch, and cassette.

51. Which is the following is *not* acceptable for use as a surface disinfectant in a dental office?
    c. Of the agents listed, glutaraldehydes are not acceptable for use as a surface disinfectant in a dental office.

52. Which of the following best describes an intermediate-level surface disinfectant?
    d. The intermediate-level disinfectant is for killing vegetative bacteria, most fungi, viruses, and *M. tuberculosis.*

53. What should you do before disinfecting a clinical contact surface?
    b. The surface is first precleaned and then sprayed or wiped a second time with the disinfectant to provide disinfection. Most products require 10 minutes to dry. If the surface is still wet when ready for the patient, wipe dry.

54. Which of the following terms indicates the highest level of killing power?
    a. A sporicidal is an agent that kills bacterial endospores and therefore can be called a sterilant.

55. Which of the following is *not* a clinical contact surface?
    c. Clinical contact surfaces are those areas that will be touched frequently with gloved hands during routine patient care.

56. What would you do to a clinical contact surface after removal of a plastic surface cover before the next patient?
    d. By carefully removing each cover without touching the underlying surface, the underlying surface is not contaminated. Covering surfaces is intended to replace precleaning and disinfecting between patients.

57. How often should you replace the plastic cover placed over the light handles?

    a. During treatment, these covers have been contaminated and must be changed after each patient.

58. Which of the following can kill bacterial spores, tuberculosis, and viruses?

    c. According to the CDC, disinfectants are categorized according to their microbial spectrum of activity. High level disinfectants destroy all microorganisms including tuberculosis and viruses but not necessarily high numbers of bacterial spores.

59. You should *not* use which of the following as a cover barrier for a bracket table?

    b. Surface covers should be impervious to fluids to keep microorganisms in saliva, blood, or other liquids from soaking through to the contact surface. Plastic-backed paper is acceptable, but not paper sheets alone.

60. Which of the following is the major disadvantage of using bleach as a surface disinfectant?

    d. Products such as bleach used as surface disinfectants can damage fabrics and metal surfaces, and its activity is reduced in the presence of organic material.

61. Which of the following best describes the Spaulding Classification System?

    b. The CDC categorizes patient care items as critical, semicritical, and noncritical based on the potential risks of infection during use of the items. These categories are referred to as the Spaulding Classification System.

62. What is the maximum acceptable level of bacteria in dental unit water as recommended by the CDC?

    c. The EPA standard for the microbial quality of drinking or potable water is no more than a total of 500 CFU/ml (colony-forming units per milliliter).

63. Which of the following best defines the term *potable water?*

    c. The EPA defines potable water as drinking water.

64. How often does the CDC recommend flushing of dental unit water lines?

    a. The CDC recommends discharging water and air for a minimum of 20 to 30 seconds after each patient from any dental device connected to the dental water system that enters the patient's mouth.

65. What should you do before changing or cleaning a vacuum line trap?

    d. It is recommended that, before changing or cleaning a vacuum line trap a detergent or detergent-disinfectant be evacuated through the system.

66. Patient-to-patient cross-contamination may occur when a patient closes his or her lips around which of the following?

    b. Research has shown that previously suctioned fluids might be retracted into the patient's mouth when a seal around the saliva ejector is created, causing a type of "suck back" or reverse flow in the vacuum line that might allow the contents to reach the patient's mouth.

67. Which of the following is a disadvantage of using disposable items?

    c. Disposables pose disadvantages, including the possibility of less efficient operation than the reusable counterpart, increased expense, and the addition of nonbiodegradable materials to the environment on disposal.

68. Patient care instruments are categorized into various classifications. Into which classification would instruments such as blood pressure cuffs, pulse oximeter, and stethoscope be placed?

    c. These items would be categorized as noncritical instruments as they would not be in contact with saliva or other potentially infectious materials.

69. Ideally, when should you disinfect an impression?

a. The impression is rinsed thoroughly at chairside and placed into a zippered plastic bag containing an appropriate disinfectant.

70. You should not use which of the following to disinfect a full denture prior to sending it off to the dental lab?

c. Any prosthesis taken from the oral cavity and being sent to the laboratory should be cleaned and disinfected with an EPA-registered disinfectant having at least an intermediate level of activity (tuberculocidal claim). Quaternary ammonium compounds do not meet these criteria.

71. Air suction motors on dental lathes should produce an air velocity of at least:

b. To avoid the spread of infection while using the dental lathe, the air-suction motor should be capable of producing an air velocity of at least 200 ft/min.

72. What should you do if your x-ray positioners cannot be autoclaved?

c. For maximum protection, x-ray positioners that cannot be autoclaved should be soaked in a high-level disinfectant.

73. What should you do when using a daylight loader?

d. The only aseptic way to use a daylight loader is to insert only disinfected or unsoiled film packs (those that have been placed in pouches) into the unit and to use powder-free gloves.

74. Which of the following is an example of regulated medical waste?

c. Regulated waste is infectious medical waste that requires special handling, neutralization, and disposal. Used anesthetic needles fall into this category.

75. A sharps container is an example of a(n):

c. Engineering and work practice controls are used to minimize or eliminate exposure. The use of a sharps container is an example of engineering controls.

76. Which of the following is *not* a recognized type of regulated medical waste?

c. Used PPEs are not a type of related medical waste. The other items listed all fall under regulated waste as they are potential infectious medical waste that require special handling and disposal.

77. Regulated medical waste comprises what percentage of a dental office's total waste?

a. Infectious waste is a small amount of the medical waste that has shown the capability of transmitting an infectious disease and ranges at 3% or less.

78. What should you do if the outside of a biohazard bag becomes contaminated?

d. If the outside of a biohazard bag becomes contaminated, simply place it inside another biohazard bag.

79. How would you properly sterilize filled sharps containers in-house?

d. In-house stylization of filled sharps containers requires that the container must be autoclavable and that the container vents be left open.

80. What federal agency requires employers to inform employees of their risk and to offer free the hepatitis B vaccine?

b. In the OSHA Bloodborne Pathogens Standard, the employer is informed of the conditions under which the hepatitis B vaccine is to be offered to employees.

81. According to OSHA, which of the following is most effective in protecting employees while at work?
   b. Engineering controls are measures designed to remove the bloodborne pathogens and chemical hazards from the workplace.

82. Which of the following is a specific eye, mouth, other mucous membrane, nonintact skin, or parenteral contact with blood or other potentially infectious materials that results from the performance of an employee's duties?
   c. An exposure incident means a specific eye, mouth, or other mucous membrane, nonintact skin, or parenteral contact with blood or other potentially infectious materials that results from the performance of an employee's duties as defined in the OSHA Bloodborne Pathogens Standard.

83. After initial training, how often must employees receive training concerning the OSHA Bloodborne Pathogens Standard?
   c. In accordance with the OSHA Bloodborne Pathogens Standard, after initial training the employees must receive further training at least annually.

84. According the Spaulding Classification System, dental explorers are:
   a. The explorer is a critical instrument in that it may penetrate soft tissue, contact bone, or enter into contact with the bloodstream or other normally sterile tissue of the mouth.

85. Why is it important to dry instrument packages inside the sterilizer after the end of a sterilization cycle?
   a. Handling wet packages of instruments can cause them to tear and thus become contaminated. Exposing wet packages to the environment outside the sterilizer can cause wicking, a process that allows bacteria and fungi to penetrate wet sterilization paper.

86. How would you minimize corrosion of carbon steel instruments during sterilization?
   d. The use of dry heat or unsaturated chemical vapor sterilization will prevent carbon steel instruments from rusting.

87. What is the purpose of the Hazard Communication Standard?
   b. The hazard communication program has been developed to ensure that employers and employees know about work hazards and know how to protect themselves from potential injuries from hazardous materials.

88. Who provides MSDS?
   d. The manufacturer of the chemical product is responsible to provide an MSDS for each product.

89. How many sections are there in an MSDS?
   d. On each MSDS, there are nine different sections providing data and information about the product.

90. What must you have for every hazardous chemical in your work environment?
   a. For each hazardous chemical product used in the dental office, there must be an MSDS on file.

91. There is a diamond-shaped symbol on the bottle of a chemical in your office. Its red-colored section has the number four written inside. What does this mean?
   d. This symbol is the identification code for flammability and indicates that the material will rapidly or completely vaporize at atmospheric pressure and normal ambient temperature or, when readily dispersed in air, will burn readily.

92. According to the Hazard Communication Standard, employees must receive training at the time of their initial assignment and then:
   b. The HazCom Standard requires training of an employee at the initial hiring and also upon the introduction of a new hazardous material or condition.

93. You should *not* consider which of the following to be a hazardous chemical?
    c. Some chemicals are exempt from the HazCom Standard including, but not limited, to aspirin.

94. Who designates a chemical as being hazardous?
    b. The EPA is the agency that designates which chemicals are hazardous.

95. A hospital level disinfectant is the same as a(n):
    b. The EPA-registered hospital disinfectants are categorized as intermediate-level disinfectants.

96. What is the goal of infection control?
    a. The goal of infection control is to reduce the number of microorganisms that may be shared between individuals or between individuals and contaminated surfaces.

97. Which of the following procedures helps protect both a dental assistant and dental patients?
    b. The use of gloves during treatment protects the dental assistant as well as the patients.

98. You must remove which of the following when temporarily leaving a seated patient?
    c. When a dental health care worker leaves the treatment room temporarily, the gloves must be removed and, when returning to chairside, the hands must be rewashed and regloved. The alternative to this option is to wear overgloves when leaving the treatment room.

99. Which of the following is the least desirable method for cleaning dental instruments?
    b. To protect the dental health care worker during instrument processing, protective utility gloves should be used, but instruments should not be scrubbed by hand. Instruments should be mechanically cleaned.

100. Use of liquid sterilants, such as glutaraldehyde, is restricted to what type of reusable items?
    c. Liquid sterilants are used for reusable items that cannot be heat sterilized.

Contacts

NATIONAL CONTACTS

American Dental Association
211 East Chicago Avenue
Chicago, Illinois 60611-2678
312-440-2500
www.ada.org

American Dental Assistants Association
35 East Wacker Drive
Suite 1730
Chicago, Illinois 60601-2211
312-541-1550
www.dentalassistant.org

The Dental Assisting National Board, Inc. (DANB)
444 North Michigan Avenue
Suite 900
Chicago, Illinois 60611-3985
1-800-FOR-DANB or 312-642-3368
www.danb.org

STATE CONTACTS

Board of Dental Examiners of Alabama
www.dentalboard.org
205-985-7267

Alaska State Board of Dental Examiners
www.dced.state.ak.us/occ/pden.htm
907-465-2542

Arizona State Board of Dental Examiners
www.azdentalboard.org
602-242-1492

Arkansas State Board of Dental Examiners
www.asbde.org
501-682-2085

California/Committee on Dental Auxiliaries
www.comda.ca.gov
916-263-2595

Colorado State Board of Dental Examiners
www.dora.state.co.us/dental
303-894-7758

Connecticut State Dental Commission/Department of Public Health
www.dph.state.ct.us/bch/oralhealth/index
860-509-8388

Delaware Department of Health
www.dpr.delaware.gov/boards/dental/index.shtml
302-744-4700

Department of Health-District of Columbia Board of Dentistry
www.dchealth.dc.gov
202-724-4900

Florida Board of Dentistry
www.doh.state.fl.us/mqa/dentistry/
850-245-4474

Georgia Board of Dentistry
www.sos.state.ga.us/plb/dentistry
478-207-2445

Hawaii State Board of Dental Examiners
www.hawaii.gov/dcca/areas/pvl/boards/dentist
808-586-3000

Idaho State Board of Dentistry
www2.state.id.us/isbd
208-334-2369

Illinois State Board of Dentistry
www.idfpr.com
217-782-8556

Indiana State Department of Health
http://www.in.gov/pla/blandc/isbd/
317-233-7565

Iowa Board of Dental Examiners
www.state.ia.us/dentalboard
515-281-5157

Kansas Dental Board
www.accesskansas.org/kdb
785-296-6400

Kentucky Board of Dentistry
www.dentistry.ky.gov
502-429-7280

Louisiana State Board of Dentistry
www.lsbd.org
504-568-8574

Maine Board of Dental Examiners
www.mainedental.org
207-287-3333

Maryland State Board of Dental Examiners
www.dhmh.state.md.us/dental
410-402-8500

Massachusetts Board of Registration in Dentistry
www.mass.gov/dpl/boards/dn
617-973-0971

Michigan Board of Dentistry
www.michigan.gov/healthlicense
517-335-0918

Minnesota Board of Dentistry
www.dentalboard.state.mn.us
612-617-2250

Mississippi State Board of Dental Examiners
www.msbde.state.ms.us
601-944-9622

Missouri Dental Board
pr.mo.gov/dental.asp
573-751-0040

Montana Board of Dentistry
www.discoveringmontana.com/dli/den
406-841-2390

Nebraska Board of Dentistry – Credentialing Division
www.hhs.state.ne.us/crl/medical/dent/dentist/dentist.htm
402-471-2118

Nevada State Board of Dental Examiners
www.nvdentalboard.org/
1-800-DDS-EXAM or 702-486-7044

New Hampshire Board of Dental Examiners
www.state.nh.us/dental
603-271-4561

New Jersey State Board of Dentistry
www.state.nj.us/lps/ca/medical/dentistry.htm
973-504-6405

New Mexico Board of Dental Health Care
www.rld.state.nm.us/Dental/index.html
505-476-4680

New York State Board for Dentistry
www.op.nysed.gov/dent.htm
518-474-3817

North Carolina State Board of Dental Examiners
www.ncdentalboard.org
919-678-8223

North Dakota State Board of Dental Examiners
www.nddentalboard.org
701-258-8600

Ohio State Dental Board
www.dental.ohio.gov
614-466-2580

Oklahoma State Board of Dentistry
www.dentist.state.ok.us
405-524-9037

Oregon Board of Dentistry
www.oregondentistry.org
503-229-5520

Pennsylvania State Board of Dentistry
www.dos.state.pa.us/dent
717-783-7162

Rhode Island State Board of Examiners in Dentistry
www.health.ri.gov/hsr/professions/dental.php
401-222-1392

South Carolina State Board of Dentistry
www.llr.state.sc.us/pol/dentistry/default.htm
803-896-4599

South Dakota State Board of Dentistry
www.state.sd.us/doh/dentistry
605-224-1282

Tennessee Board of Dentistry
http://health.state.tn.us/Boards/Dentistry
800-778-4123 x24721

Texas State Board of Dental Examiners
www.tsbde.state.tx.us
512-463-6400

Utah Dentists and Dental Hygienists Licensing Board
www.dopl.utah.gov/licensing/dentistry.html
801-530-6740

Vermont State Board of Dental Examiners
www.vtprofessionals.org/opr1/dentists
802-828-2390

Virginia Board of Dentistry
www.dhp.virginia.gov/dentistry/default.htm
804-662-9906

Washington State Dental Health Care Authority
https://fortress.wa.gov/doh/hpqa1/hps3/Dental/
    default.htm
360-236-4822

West Virginia Board of Dental Examiners
www.wvdentalboard.org
877-914-8266

Wisconsin Dentistry Examining Board
drl.wi.gov/boards/den/index.htm
608-266-2811

Wyoming Board of Dental Examiners
plboards.state.wy.us/dental/index.asp
307-777-6529

Bibliography/ Suggested Readings

Listed below are a series of references used as resources to create the examinations. You may find it helpful to review these books as you proceed to prepare for a credentialing exam or to use for future reference:

1. Aiken TD: *Legal & Ethical Issues in Health Occupations,* 2e, St. Louis, Saunders, 2008.

2. Anusavice KJ: *Phillips' Science of Dental Materials,* 11e, St. Louis, Saunders, 2003.

3. Ash MM, Jr., Nelson S: *Wheeler's Dental Anatomy, Physiology and Occlusion,* 8e, St. Louis, Saunders, 2003.

4. Avery JK, Chiego DJ: *Essentials of Oral Histology and Embryology: A Clinical Approach,* 3e, St. Louis, Mosby, 2006.

5. Bath-Balogh M, Fehrenbach MJ: *Illustrated Dental Embryology, Histology and Anatomy,* 2e, St. Louis, Saunders, 2006.

6. Beemsterboer PL: *Ethics and Law in Dental Hygiene,* St. Louis, Saunders, 2002.

7. Bennett J, Rosenberg M: *Medical Emergencies in Dentistry,* St. Louis, Saunders, 2002.

8. Bird DL, Robinson DS: *Torres and Ehrlich Modern Dental Assisting,* 9e, St. Louis, Saunders, 2009.

9. Boyd LB: *Dental Instruments: A Pocket Guide,* 3e, St. Louis, Saunders, 2009.

10. Brand RW, Isselhard DE: *Anatomy of Orofacial Structures,* 7e, St. Louis, Mosby, 2003.

11. Burt BA, Eklund SA: *Dentistry, Dental Practice and the Community,* 6e, St. Louis, Saunders, 2005.

12. Cappelli DP, Mobley CC: *Prevention in Clinical Oral Health Care,* St. Louis, Mosby, 2008.

13. Centers for Disease Control and Prevention, *Guidelines for Infection Control in Dental Healthcare Settings – 2003, MMWR 52*(RR-17):1-68, 2003, also available at: *www.cdc.gov/mmwr/PDF/rr/rr5217.pdf*

14. Centers for Disease Control and Prevention and the Healthcare Infection Control Practices Advisory Committee (HICPAC), *Guidelines for Environmental Infection Control in Healthcare Facilities,* available at: *www.cdc.gov/ncidod/dhqp/gl_environinfection.html*

15. Clark M, Brunick A: *Handbook of Nitrous Oxide and Oxygen Sedation,* 3e, St. Louis, Mosby, 2008.

16. *DANB Review,* 3e, Dental Assisting National Board, Chicago.

17. Daniel SJ, Harfst SAC, Wilder R: *Mosby's Dental Hygiene: Concepts, Cases and Competencies,* 2e, St. Louis, Mosby, 2008.

18. Darby ML: *Mosby's Comprehensive Review of Dental Hygiene,* 6e, St. Louis, Mosby, 2006.

19. Darby ML, Walsh M: *Dental Hygiene Theory and Practice,* 2e, St. Louis, Saunders, 2003.

20. Davison JA: *Legal and Ethical Considerations for Dental Hygienists and Assistants,* St. Louis, Mosby, 2000.

21. Dietz, E: *Safety Standards and Infection Control for Dental Assistants,* Clifton Park, New York, 2002.

22. Fehrenbach MJ, Herring SW: *Illustrated Anatomy of the Head and Neck,* 3e, St. Louis, Saunders, 2007.

23. Finkbeiner BL, Finkbeiner CA: *Practice Management for the Dental Team,* 6e, St. Louis, Mosby, 2006.

24. Finkbeiner BL, Johnson CS: *Mosby's Comprehensive Review of Dental Assisting,* St. Louis, Mosby, 1997.

25. Frommer HH, Stabulas-Savage JJ: *Radiology for the Dental Professional,* 8e, St. Louis, Mosby, 2005.

26. Gaylor L: *The Administrative Dental Assistant,* 2e, St. Louis, Saunders, 2007.

27. Gluck GM, Morganstein WM: *Jong's Community Dental Health,* 5e, St. Louis, Mosby, 2002.

28. Guerink KV: *Community Oral Health Practice for the Dental Hygienist,* 2e, St. Louis, Saunders, 2005.

29. Hatrick CD, Eakle S, Bird WF: *Dental Materials: Clinical Applications for Dental Assistants and Dental Hygienists,* Philadelphia, Saunders, 2003.

30. Haveles EB: *Applied Pharmacology for the Dental Hygienist,* 5e, St. Louis, Mosby, 2007.

31. Hupp JR, Williams T, Firriolo FJ: *Dental Clinical Advisor,* St. Louis, Mosby, 2006.

32. Iannucci J, Howerton LJ: *Dental Radiography: Principles and Techniques,* 3e, St. Louis, Saunders, 2006.

33. Ibsen OAC, Phelan JA: *Oral Pathology for the Dental Hygienist,* 4e, St. Louis, Saunders, 2004.

34. Langlais RP: *Exercises in Oral Radiology and Interpretation,* 4e, St. Louis, Saunders, 2004.

35. Little JW, Falace D, Miller CS, Rhodus NL: *Dental Management of the Medically Compromised Patient,* 6e, St. Louis, Mosby, 2008.

36. Malamed SF: *Sedation: A Guide to Patient Management,* 4e, St. Louis, Mosby, 2003.

37. Malamed SF: *Medical Emergencies in the Dental Office,* 6e, St. Louis, Mosby, 2007.

38. Miller CH and Palenik CJ: *Infection Control & Management of Hazardous Materials for the Dental Team,* 3e, St. Louis, Mosby, 2005.

39. Mosby: *Spanish Terminology for the Dental Team,* St. Louis, Mosby, 2004.

40. Mosby: *Mosby's Dental Dictionary,* 2e, St. Louis, Mosby, 2007.

41. Mosby: *Mosby's Dental Drug Reference,* 8e, St. Louis, Mosby, 2008.

42. Nanci A: *Ten Cate's Oral Histology: Development, Structure and Function,* 7e, St. Louis, Mosby, 2008.

43. Nelson DM: *Saunders Review of Dental Hygiene,* St. Louis, Saunders, 2000.

44. Neville BW, Damm DD, Allen CM, Bouquot JE: *Oral and Maxillofacial Pathology,* 2e, St. Louis, Saunders, 2002.

45. Newman MG, Takei H, Klokkevold PR, Carranza FA: *Carranza's Clinical Periodontology,* 10e, St. Louis, Saunders, 2006.

46. Organization for Safety and Aseptic Procedures. *From Policy to Practice: OSAP's Guide to the Guidelines,* 2004, OSAP, Annapolis.

47. Perry DA, Beemsterboer PL, Taggart EJ: *Periodontology for the Dental Hygienist,* 3e, St. Louis, Saunders, 2007.

48. Phinney, DJ and Halstead, JH: *Dental Assisting a Comprehensive Approach,* 3e, 2008.

49. Powers JM, Wataha JC: *Dental Materials: Properties and Manipulation,* 8e, St. Louis, Mosby, 2008.

50. Regezi JA, Sciubba JJ, Jordan RCK: *Oral Pathology: Clinical Pathologic Correlations,* 5e, St. Louis, Saunders, 2008.

51. Robinson DS, Bird DL: *Essentials of Dental Assisting,* 4e, St. Louis, Elsevier, 2007.

52. Rose LF, Mealey BL, Genco RJ, Cohen DW: *Periodontics: Medicine, Surgery and Implants,* St. Louis, Saunders, 2004.

53. Samaranayake LP: *Essential Microbiology for Dentistry,* 3e, St. Louis, Saunders, 2006.

54. Sapp JP, Eversole LR, Wysocki GW: *Contemporary Oral and Maxillofacial Pathology,* 2e, St. Louis, Mosby, 2004.

55. Stegeman CA, Davis JR: *The Dental Hygienist's Guide to Nutritional Care,* 2e, St. Louis, Saunders, 2004.

56. United States Department of Labor, Occupational Safety and Health Administration, 29 CFR Part 1910.1030. Occupational Exposure to Bloodborne Pathogens; Needlesticks and Other Sharps Injuries; Final Rule. *Federal Register* 2001; 66:5317–25. As amended from and includes 29 CFR Part 1910.1030. Occupational Exposure to Bloodborne Pathogens; Final Rule. *Federal Register* 1991; 56:64174–82, available at *www.osha.gov/SLTC/dentistry/index.html*

57. United States Department of Labor, Occupational Safety and Health Administration, 29 CFR 1910.1030. Hazard Communications; Final Rule. *Federal Register* 59:6126-6184, 1994, also available at: *www.osha.gov/SLTC/hazardcommunications/index.html*

Figure Credits

Test 1 General Chairside

Figure corresponding to question 2 from Finkbeiner B and Finkbeiner C: *Practice Management for the Dental Team,* 6e, St. Louis, 2006, Mosby.

Figures corresponding to questions 30-32, 58, 64, 68, 79, 80 from Bird D and Robinson D: *Torres and Ehrlich Modern Dental Assisting,* 9e, St. Louis, 2009, Saunders.

Figures corresponding to questions 85 and 86, courtesy of Miltex, Inc, York, Pennsylvania.

Test 1 Radiation Health and Safety

Figures corresponding to questions 2, 56, 59-68, 72, 99 from Iannucci J and Jansen Howerton L: *Dental Radiography: Principles and Techniques,* 3e, St. Louis, 2006, Saunders.

Test 2 General Chairside

Figures corresponding to questions 23-29, 72-73, 79, 89-90 from Bird D and Robinson D: *Torres and Ehrlich Modern Dental Assisting,* 9e, St. Louis, 2009, Saunders.

Figure corresponding to question 46 from Finkbeiner B and Johnson C: *Mosby's Comprehensive Dental Assisting: A Clinical Approach,* St. Louis, 1995, Mosby.

Figures corresponding to questions 53-56 from Boyd L: *Dental Instruments: A Pocket Guide,* 3e, St. Louis, in press, Saunders.

Test 2 Radiation Health and Safety

Figures corresponding to questions 1, 34, and 66 from Frommer H and Stabulas-Savage J: *Radiology for the Dental Professional,* 8e, St. Louis, 2005, Mosby.

Figures corresponding to questions 2, 3, 42-45, 67-70, 73, 74, 93-100 from Iannucci J and Jansen Howerton L: *Dental Radiography: Principles and Techniques,* 3e, St. Louis, 2006, Saunders.

Test 3 General Chairside

Figure corresponding to question 24 from Finkbeiner B and Johnson C: *Mosby's Comprehensive Dental Assisting: A Clinical Approach,* St. Louis, 1995, Mosby.

Figures corresponding to questions 30 and 31 from Boyd L: *Dental Instruments: A Pocket Guide,* 3e, St. Louis, 2009, Saunders.

Figures corresponding to questions 4, 6, 7, 9, 46, 49, 59, 64, 65, and 87 from Bird D and Robinson D: *Torres and Ehrlich Modern Dental Assisting,* 9e, St. Louis, 2009, Saunders.

Test 3 Radiation Health and Safety

Figure corresponding to question 61 from Frommer H and Stabulas-Savage J: *Radiology for the Dental Professional,* 8e, St. Louis, 2005, Mosby.

Figures corresponding to questions 31-34, 36, 40, 41, 60, 63, 70-73, and 81 from Iannucci J and Jansen Howerton L: *Dental Radiography: Principles and Techniques,* 3e, St. Louis, 2006, Saunders.

FAZIE — 647 997 5184

Tony — 416 802 5184